50 All Natural
Body, Skin, and Hair Recipes

Quick, Simple and Easy Recipes to Enhance the Beauty of your Body, Skin and Hair!

Disclaimer

The remedies mentioned here should not be used if they alter or substitute with your medical therapy without taking your doctor's advice. For a certain health problems, consult your physician first before using the recipes in this eBook.

Always check with your physician to avoid any adverse effects that could rise from the usage of these recipes if you have an existing medical condition, or if you are pregnant or nursing.

Some herbs can also interact with your medical prescriptions including antidepressants and the Pill. Furthermore, if thinking of using any of the skin balms, always do a 24-hour skin/patch test before using to avoid any allergic reactions from the ingredients. It is understood that the reader claims responsibility for their own actions.

All information, recipes and ideas presented here are for educational purposes only. The author cannot be held responsible for any personal or commercial damage caused by misinterpretation of information or improper use of the details in this book.

Contents

Disclaimer 2

Natural Home Remedies for Beautiful Hair 7

  Yogurt for Dull Hair 7

    Remedies 7

      a.   *Use of Plain Yogurt:* 7

      b.   *Yogurt, Apple Cider and Honey* 8

      c.   *Yogurt and Coconut oil* 8

  Honey to Cure Dry and Damaged Hair 9

    Remedies: 9

      a.   *Just Honey for Damaged and Dry Hair* 9

      b.   *Honey and Avocado* 9

      c.   Honey and Egg Yolk 10

  Corn Starch to Reduce Oiliness of Hair 12

  Remedies: 12

      a.   *Cornstarch for Greasy Hair* 12

  Avocado to Cure Frizzy Hair 14

    Remedies: 14

      a.   *Avocado for Frizzy or Damp Hair:* 14

      b.   *Avocado and Olive Oil* 15

      c.   *Avocado and Peppermint Oil* 15

  Onion Juice for Strong Hair 17

    Remedies: 17

      a.   *Use of Onion Juice for Stronger Hair* 17

      b.   *Onion Juice and Honey* 18

      c.   *Onion juice and Egg Yolk* 18

  Egg Yolk to Cure Hair Loss 20

    Remedies: 20

      a.   *Use of Egg yolk to Cure Hair Fall* 20

      b.   *Egg Yolk, Olive Oil and Honey* 21

      c.   *Egg Yolk and Lime Juice* 22

  Fenugreek Seeds to Cure Severe Hair Loss 23

Remedies: 23

   a.   Fenugreek Seed Paste: 23

   b.   Fenugreek Oil and Yogurt: 24

   c.   Hot Oil Massage 24

   d.   Fenugreek Leaves and Apple Cider 25

Potato Juice for Hair Growth 26

How to Make Potato Juice 26

   Remedies 27

   a.   *Potato Juice for Hair* 27

   b.   *Potato Juice, Honey and Egg Mask for Hair* 27

Henna Powder for Shiny Hair 29

   Remedies: 29

   a.   Henna and Honey 29

   b.   Henna, Tea and Coffee for Conditioning and Coloring 30

   c.   Henna and Orange Juice 31

   d.   Henna, Shikakai and Gooseberry powder 32

Aloe Vera for Longer and Stronger Hair 33

   Remedies: 33

   a.   Aloe Vera Gel For Hair Growth and Strength: 33

   b.   Hibiscus Flower Powder and Aloe Gel for Hair Loss 34

   c.   Lemon Juice and Aloe Gel for Oily Hair 35

Orange Juice to Get Rid Of the Dandruff and Itchy Scalp 36

   Remedies: 36

   a.   Apple and Orange Juice Tonic for Hair Growth 36

   b.   Orange Peel Paste for Hair Growth 37

Natural Home Remedies for Flawless Skin 38

Baking Soda to Get Rid of the Blemish Scars 38

Neem Tree Leaves To Reduce Acne and Blemishes 39

   Remedies: 39

   Neem Tree Leaves Paste and Oil as a Cure for Blemishes 39

Milk and Cucumber Mask to Get Rid of the Oily Skin and Blemishes 40

   Remedy: 40

a.   Milk and Cucumber Mask For Blemishes and Oil Control: 40

b.   Cucumber Toner for Oil Control: 40

Honey Treatment to Get Rid of the Dark Spots and Blemishes: 41

Remedies: 41

Honey and Lemon to Cure Dark Spot and Prevent Blemishes: 41

Turmeric Powder and Milk Cream to Lighten Your Skin Tone 42

Remedies: 42

Turmeric, Saffron and Milk Cream 42

Mud Mask to reduce Oil from Face 43

Remedies: 43

Fuller's Earth Mask 43

Cabbage Toner and Green Tea to Reduce Oil on Skin 44

Remedies: 44

Cabbage Toner 44

Green Tea Toner 45

Egg White Mask to Reduce Wrinkles 46

Remedies: 46

How to Prepare Egg Mask: 46

Remove Black and Whiteheads with Nutmeg 47

Remedies 47

Nutmeg Paste 47

Tomato Pulp to Remove Whiteheads 48

Remedies: 48

Tomato Paste and Tonic to Cure Whiteheads 48

Banana Mask to Deal with Dry and Patchy Skin 49

Remedy: 49

Banana Mask 49

Use of Shea Butter and Butter Milk to Moisturize Skin 50

Remedy: 50

Butter milk and Shea Butter Moisturizer: 50

Natural Home Remedies for Maintaining a Fit and Beautiful Body 51

Apricot and Avocado Scrub for Natural Shine on Body 51

Remedies: 51

Apricot and Avocado Scrub Made at Home: 51

Quinoa to Oxidize blood and Reduce Excess Weight 53

Remedy: 53

Quinoa Tea 53

Use of Honey and Lemon to Keep Your Body Weight in Check 54

Remedy: 54

Lemon and Honey Tea 54

Oatmeal to Reduce Cholesterol and Living a Healthy and Fit life 55

Remedies: 55

a.   Oat Meal, Honey and Pumpkin 55

b.   Oat Meal Yogurt and Raspberries 55

c.   Oat Meal, Coconut and Milk 56

Use of Olive Oil to Reduce Weight 57

Remedy 57

Olive Oil an Active Weight Reducing Agent 57

Adding A Little Cinnamon to Keep the Body in Shape 58

Remedy 58

Cinnamon Tea: 58

Use of Cabbage for Flat Tummy 59

Remedy: 59

Cabbage Soup to Reduce 59

Water Melon Diet to Keep Those Extra Pounds Away 60

Remedy: 60

Watermelon to Effectively Lose Weight 60

Conclusion: 61

Natural Home Remedies for Beautiful Hair

Yogurt for Dull Hair

Yogurt can account for an extremely healthy breakfast, lunch or dinner. But did you know you can use yogurt or curd to bring life back to your dull and dry hair? Exactly! Your hair loves yogurt, just as much as you do.

Yogurt is being used as an integral ingredient in most of the products for dull and dry hair available in the market. But make it a point that, no chemical product can substitute the benefit that using all natural product will do.

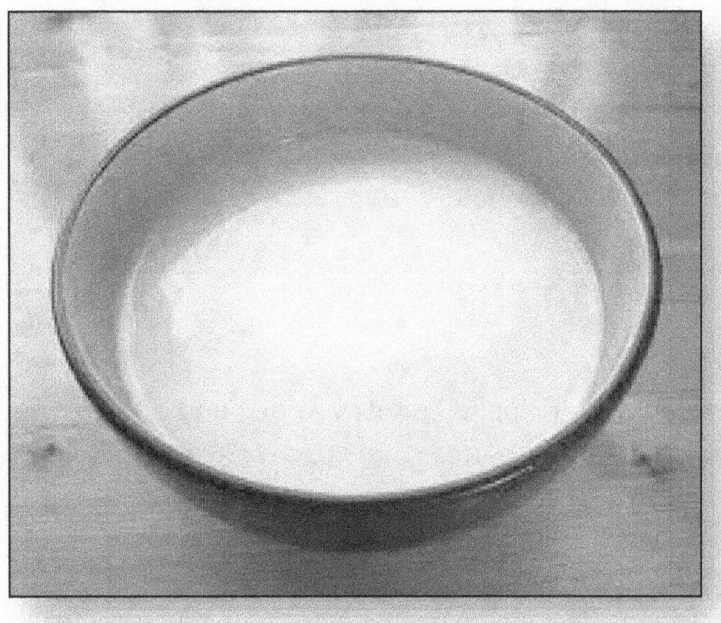

You can apply yogurt or curd to your hair independently or in a combination of few other essential ingredients to cure your dull and dry hair.

Remedies

a. Use of Plain Yogurt:

The first and the easiest way to get rid of the dry hair are to moisturize your hair with yogurt. Beat the curd into a fine paste and apply it directly with fingers on your scalp. Apply a good amount of yogurt and massage gently for 10 minutes at least. Give it a rest for 30 minutes and then you can wash your hair with any mild shampoo.
You can repeat the procedure once or twice a week.

b. Yogurt, Apple Cider and Honey

Apple cider vinegar is known for bringing back the shine and softness to hair. Honey and curd moisturizes your hair from the core making them appear, healthy, shiny and full of life.

Ingredients:

½ Cup Yogurt

1 Tablespoon of Apple Cider Vinegar

2Tablespoon of Honey

Process:

Mix all the ingredients and beat them until they start to look like a paste. Apply the mixture to your scalp and massage gently apply the remnant of the mixture on your hair and cover them properly.

Make sure that you don't over use the apple cider vinegar. Apple cider is a bit acidic in nature. It has no adverse effects on your hair, however they can cause a burning sensation on your scalp if used alone or greater quantity than it is prescribed.

Let the mixture stay in your hair for about half an hour then wash your hair with any mild shampoo.

c. Yogurt and Coconut oil

Yogurt mixed with coconut oil, if applied directly to dull and dry hair, have miraculous effects. They moisturize your hair from root to tip.

Ingredients:

2 Tablespoon of Coconut Oil

½ Cup of Yogurt

Process:

Make a fine paste of the ingredient and apply directly to your hair. Massage your scalp and absorb the ingredients in it. Let it stay in your hair for about half an hour and then you can wash your hair with warm water and any good fruit shampoo.

Honey to Cure Dry and Damaged Hair

When it comes to dry and damaged hair skin, honey is your go-to-solution of the problem. Honey has natural ability and an essential ingredient like humectants which draws moisture to the surface of your scalp from the environment. Providing them the hydration they need to appear shiny, beautiful and healthy.

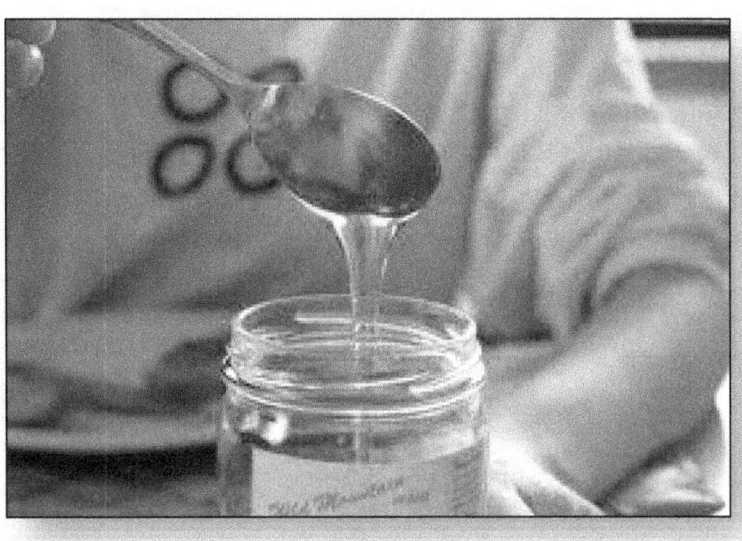

Honey also provides your hair the strength to grow and nourishes your hair from root to tip. Healthy hair accounts for the natural beauty in you, after all. If you wish to have longer hair, than these remedies are for you.

You can either directly apply honey to your or in the combination of other ingredients. Either way it is going to yield great results.

Remedies:

a. Just Honey for Damaged and Dry Hair

The easiest way to cure the dryness of your hair is by applying honey directly to your hair. Take 2-3 tablespoon of honey; add enough water to dilute honey into a solution. Apply this solution directly on your scalp and massage thoroughly.

Let the solution stay in your hair for almost half an hour. Wash your hair with any good egg shampoo.

b. Honey and Avocado

For extremely dry hair you can always add other ingredients which are known for curing dry and damaged hair along with honey, for instance Avocado. Honey attracts the moisture from the environment and secures them in your hair.

Ingredients:

½ Avocado

3 tablespoon of honey

Water to dilute Honey

Process:

Dilute honey by adding water to it and then add ½ avocado by crushing and grinding it into small pieces. Mix well and then apply the mixture on your scalp. Massage gently for 5 minutes and then let it stay in your hair for half an hour before washing your hair thoroughly. Use mild shampoo for washing your hair afterwards.

c. Honey and Egg Yolk

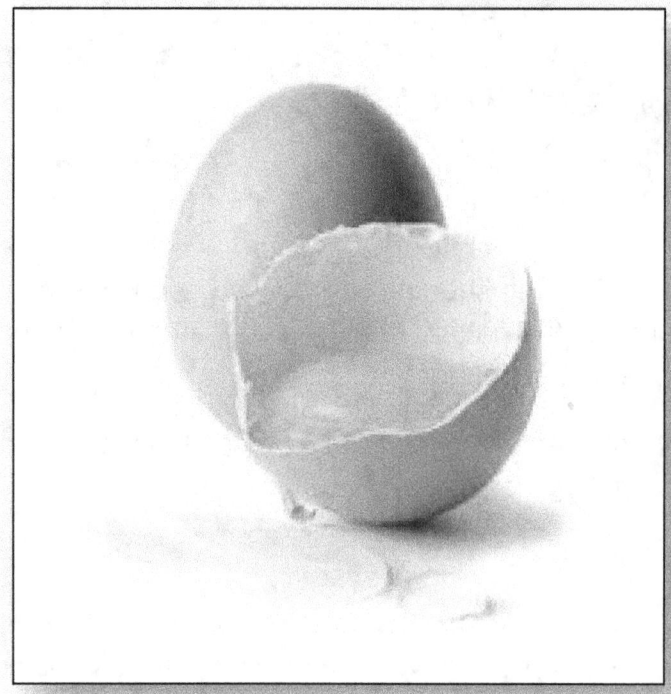

Egg yolk is full of natural proteins that your hair needs to grow. Usually dry hair gets weak and tends to break while combing. To cure dull, dry and weak hair, you need to use this remedy once or twice a week for best results.

Ingredients:

1 Egg Yolk

3 Tablespoon Honey

Process:

Beat the egg yolk and add honey to it. Make a uniform mixture of the two. Apply the mixture directly on your scalp and massage to make foam. Apply the rest of the mixture on your hair and massage for 10 minutes. Wash your thoroughly with a mild shampoo and lukewarm water.

Corn Starch to Reduce Oiliness of Hair

Some people have extra oily hair. This makes their hair look oily and grease. No one likes to have a bad hair day, especially not when you have showered and people ask, "Have you oil in your hair?"

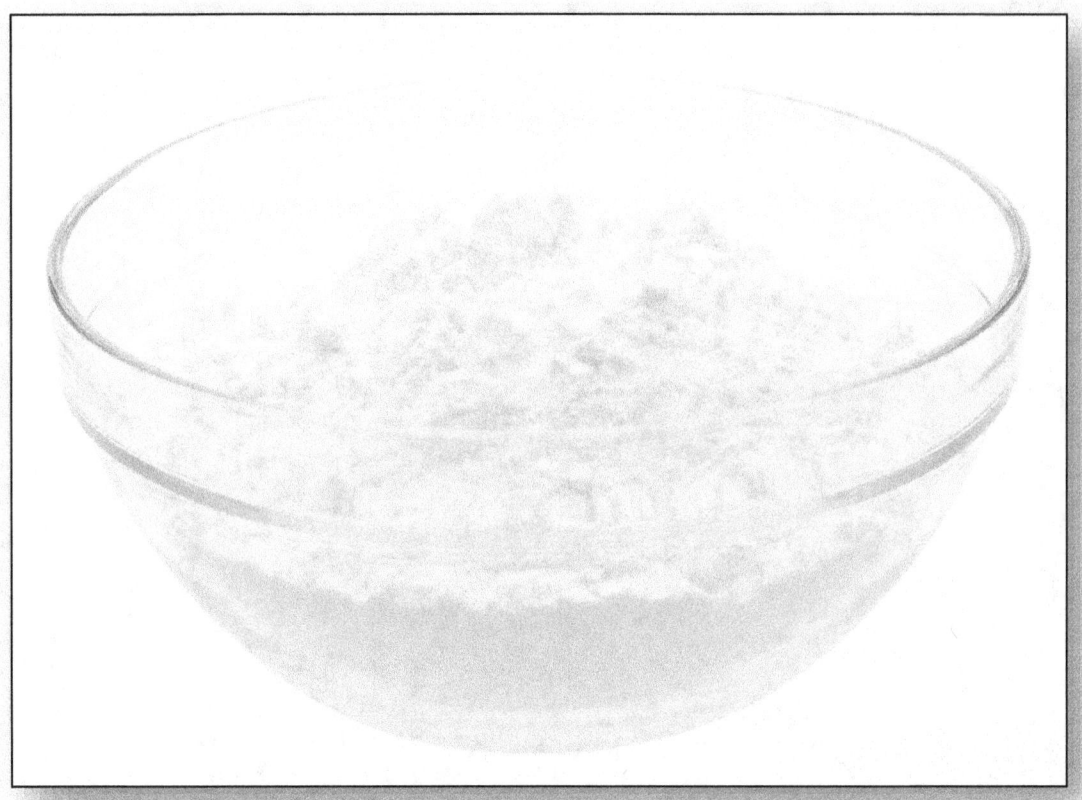

To avoid such situations all you need to do is follow some good and easy home remedies to help you in curing the oiliness of your hair.

Remedies:

a. *Cornstarch for Greasy Hair*

On the first day of your shower your hair may look really well and not so oily. You can do this on the second day of your shower or on the first day if they already feel greasy and oily.

Ingredients:

2-3 tablespoon of corn starch

Pinch of baking soda

Process:

Mix the two ingredients well and dust the mixture bit by bit onto your scalp with the help of your fingers. Massage well. Apply some on your hands and then apply thoroughly on your strands if they feel greasy. Brush your hair before going out.

You can repeat the procedure every day; it will in no way harm your hair. And even on the third and fourth day of shower your hair will feel fresh.

Avocado to Cure Frizzy Hair

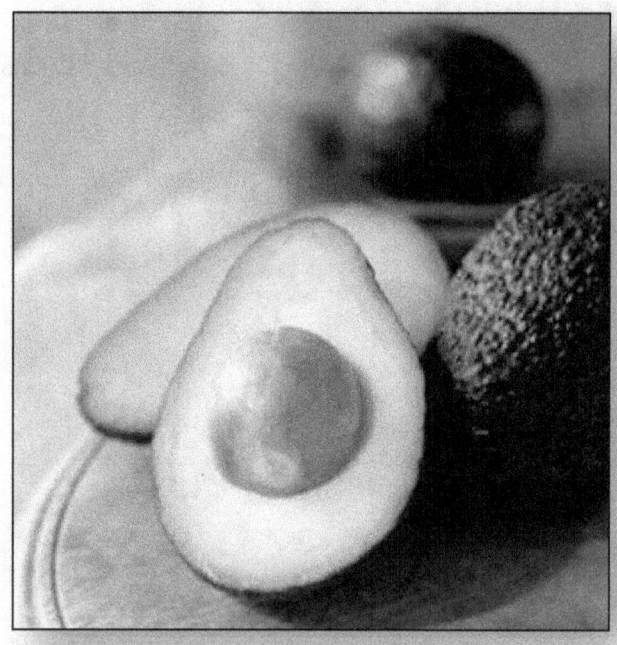

Summer is everyone's favorite season. Everyone gets to party and enjoy the bounties of the season but some time with the sunny season comes bad hair days. Most of the people complain about their hair going all Frizzy or damp and even too oily. Not really a great season for hair.

Avocado is not only essential for your personal beauty but its oils and avocado itself works like magic for damp hair. If your hair feels life less and damp than Avocado remedies will help you in revitalizing and bringing your hair back to life.

Remedies:

a. *Avocado for Frizzy or Damp Hair:*

If your hair is damp then applying avocado paste directly on to your scalp will help you in getting rid of the excess moisture in your hair and scalp. Take half avocado and make a mixture by grinding it with water. Make sure the mixture is smooth.

Apply the mixture directly to your scalp and leave it for half an hour. Wash your hair with water after wards and then with some mild shampoo.

b. Avocado and Olive Oil

Ingredients:

½ Avocado

3-4 tablespoon of Olive Oil

Water to make a paste

Process:

Grind all the ingredients and make a fine paste. Apply the fine paste with the tips of your finger on to your scalp and massage gently. Let the mixture stay on your scalp for good 30 minutes and then wash your hair thoroughly with any fruit or mild shampoo. You will see visible result after the first wash.

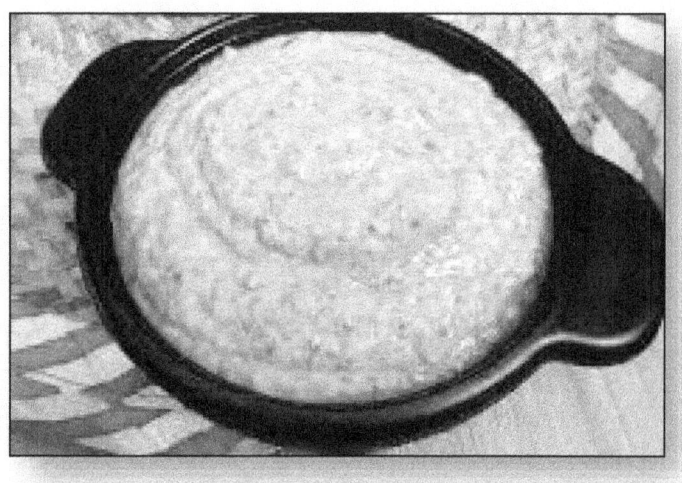

If you cover all of your hair with the avocado paste it will not only nourish your hair but will also make them soft and shiny.

c. Avocado and Peppermint Oil

Ingredients:

Half Avocado

2-3 drops of Peppermint Oil

Process:

Grind well and make a fine paste of avocado in blender. Take the mixture out in a clean bowl and add2-3 drops of peppermint oil. This oil is easily available in the market or at the nearest drug store. Mix the oil in the paste and leave it for 5 minutes. Apply the paste in your hair and massage your scalp.

The avocado will cure the frizzy hair due to the sunny weather and the essential oil will provide the nourishment they lack. You can repeat the process 2-3 times a week for best results.

Onion Juice for Strong Hair

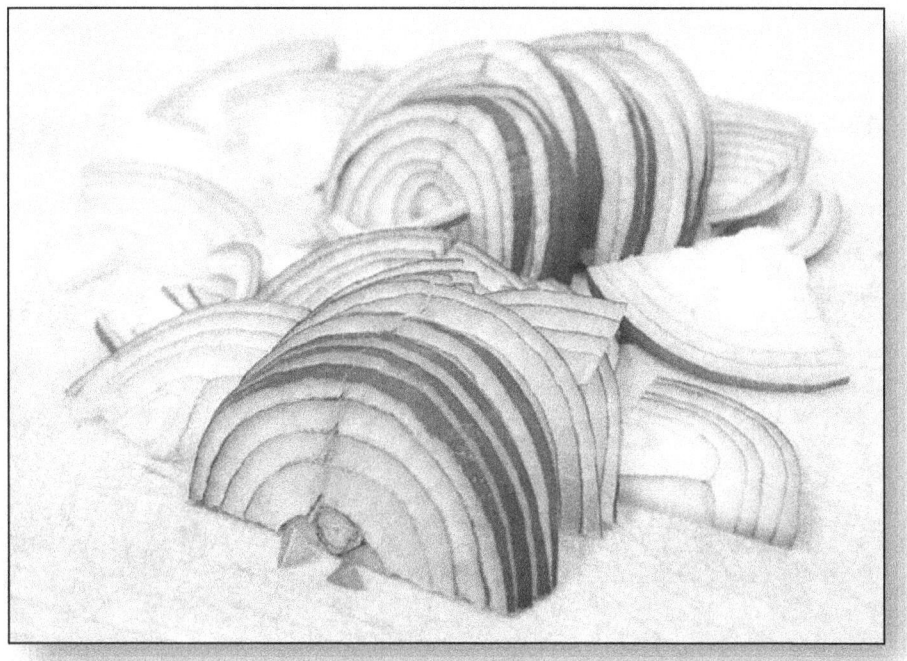

As much as we love to play with our hair, styling and combing them into fancy hairstyles, there is this one problem that keeps us from doing that –Hair fall. Our hair tends to get weak with constant styling. Your hair needs to be extremely strong if you want to twist, curl or dye them.

For long and strong hair, there are a couple of home remedies that has been among us from quite some time, for instance Onion juice. Yes, as annoying as the idea of having onion juice in your hair and having to endure its foul smell sounds. You will be actually delighted to know that all this is worth the results.

Onion juice makes the roots of your hair strong; this allows your hair to grow long. If you have a case of severe hair fall than this home remedy is for you. It will not only make your hair strong but will help in re-growth of the hair.

Remedies:

  a. *Use of Onion Juice for Stronger Hair*
Take small and red onions, 3-4 onions will be enough to make one glass juice for your hair. Chop the onions and grind them with water to make a paste. Add some more water and blend. Extract the water and put aside the remnants of onion.

Apply the juice of onion in your hair directly. And massage well. Let the juice dry and then apply some more juice. Repeat the process 5-6 times before washing your hair.

Use a shampoo with good fragrance to wash your hair afterwards to get rid of the smell on the onion form your hair.

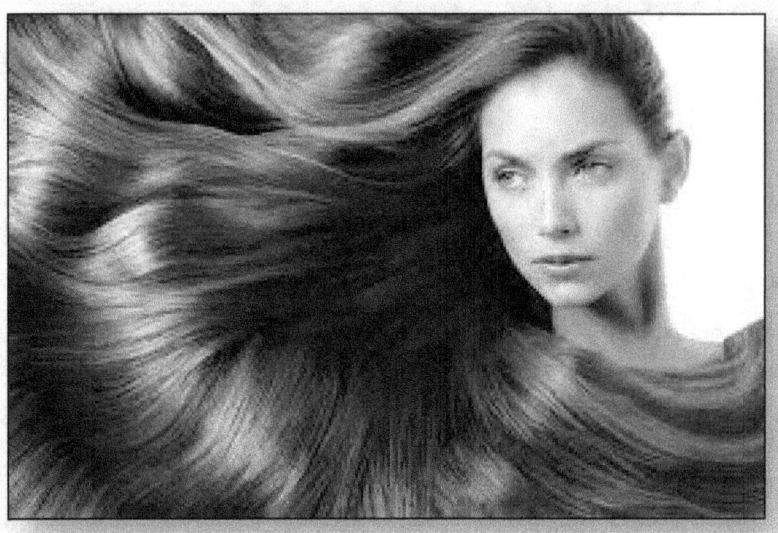

b. Onion Juice and Honey

Ingredients:

2-3 Red Onions

2Tablespoon of Honey

Water

Process:

Blend chopped onions with water make onion juice. Extract the juice form the mixture and dissolve honey in it. Apply the solution of honey and onion juice on your scalp. Allow it dry and then repeat the process. Massage well and absorb it in your scalp. Wash your hair afterwards with a mild shampoo.

c. Onion juice and Egg Yolk

Ingredients:

2-3 Red Onions

1 Egg yolk

Process:

Beat egg yolk and add it to the onion juice. Make a uniform solution and apply it to your scalp and your hair. Massage your scalp and hair in slow circular motion. Wash your hair after 15 minutes and feel the difference.

Egg Yolk to Cure Hair Loss

Hair loss is a very common problem among men and women. Everyone seems concerned that how to get rid of this major issue in their life –Hair Fall! As heart breaking is the problem is, thanks to the natural remedies curing the hair loss is not that big of an issue. All you need is consistent and sincere efforts.

No matter how much those leading shampoo companies brand they have egg and other essential ingredients in their product. The reality is nothing can be a substitute of natural products.

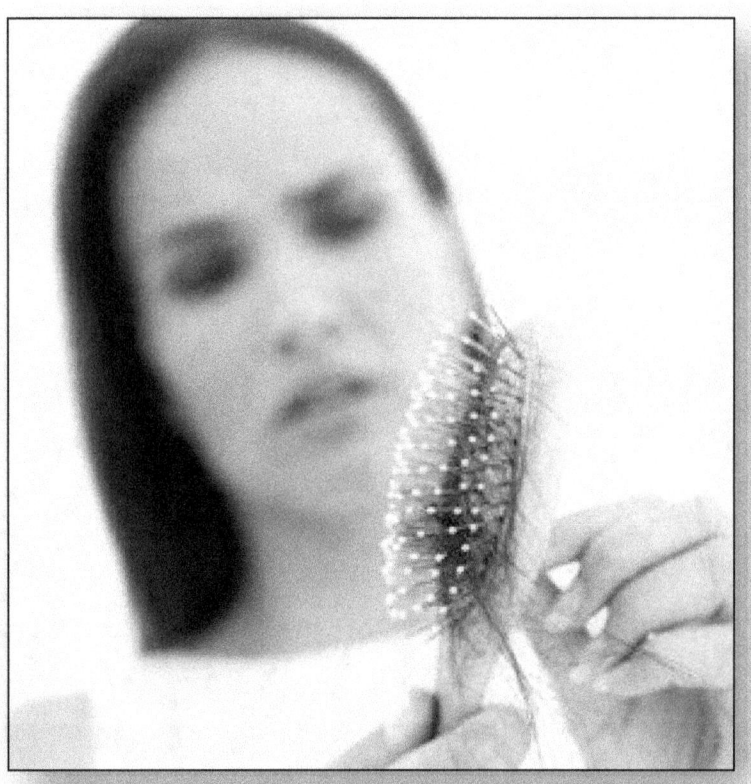

Egg yolk is being used as the key ingredient to cure hair loss. Egg yolk has vitamin A and E in abundance. These are the essential elements that your hair needs to be strong. The benefits egg yolk has to offer are not limited to curing hair loss. It actually protects your hair from harmful UV rays.

Remedies:

a. Use of Egg yolk to Cure Hair Fall

Take one or two egg yolk, depending upon the health and length of your hair. Beat them well and apply them directly on your Head. Massage your hair in circular motion like you do when you are shampooing. Wash your hair with any mild shampoo.

DO this 3-4 times in the first week, then once or twice a week after that. You will start seeing visible results in 2 weeks.

  b. Egg Yolk, Olive Oil and Honey

Ingredients:

1 Egg yolk

2 Tablespoons of Olive Oil

1 tablespoon of honey

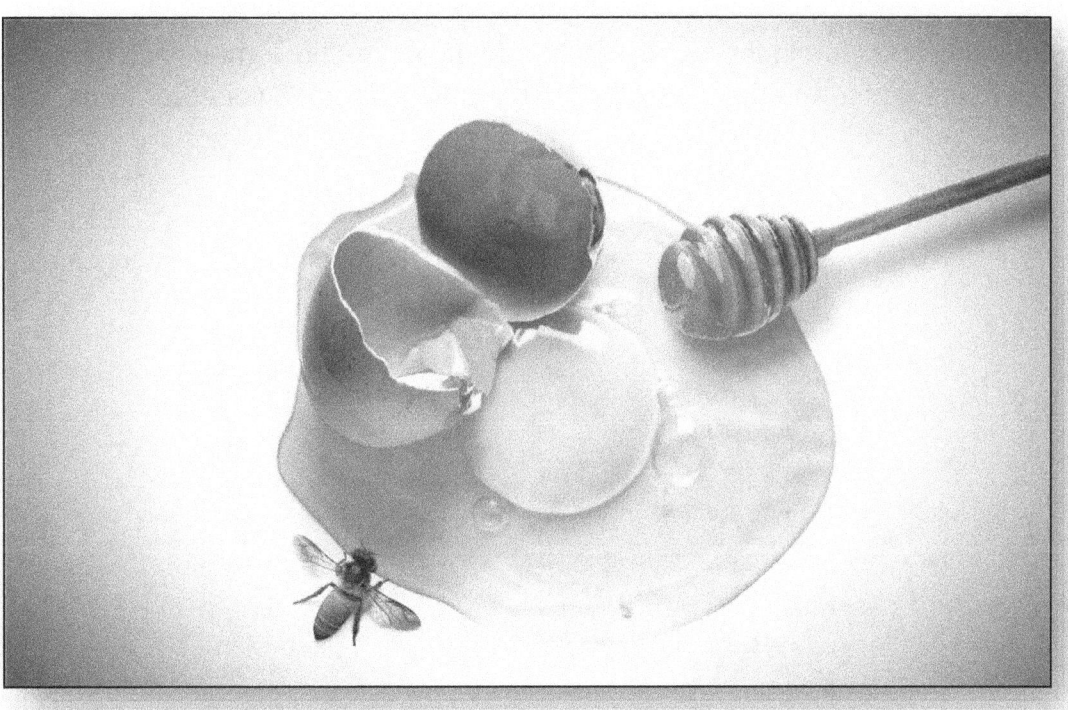

Process:

Beat the yolk, honey and add olive oil to. Beat the mixture until they form uniform consistency.

Apply the mixture on your hair and scalp like a shampoo. A little bit of leather will be formed due to the massage. Keep massaging for good 10 minutes. Wash your hair with good anti-hair fall shampoo afterwards.

c. Egg Yolk and Lime Juice

Ingredients:

1 Egg Yolk

2-3 tablespoon lime juice

Process:

Beat one egg yolk and lime juice together. Add a little water if you feel the mixture is a bit thick. Apply the whole mixture on your hair like a shampoo and massage well. The lime juice will balance the pH level of your scalp.

At times the hair loss due to the increased acidity of your scalp, lemon juice helps in curing that to prevent further hair loss. You can apply this remedy once or twice a week.

Fenugreek Seeds to Cure Severe Hair Loss

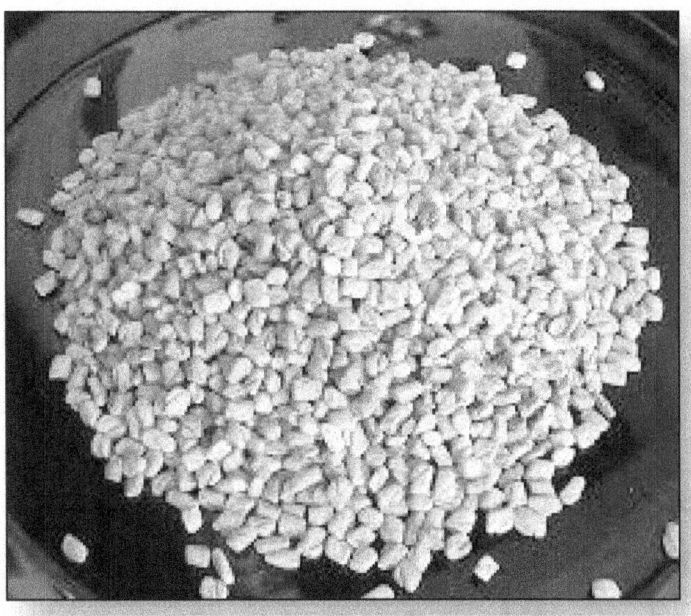

Having long and strong hair is a dream of every girl. Even men want to have strong hair to look attractive. Due to the work load, stress and environmental pollution, the problem of hair fall has increased.

Fenugreek leaves and seeds are being used to cure hair loss from quite a long time. Fenugreek seeds, leaves or even their powder can be used in several home remedies. It is a natural and effective way for hair growth.

Remedies:

a. Fenugreek Seed Paste:

Ingredients:

1 cup Fenugreek Seeds

Process:

Soak the fenugreek seeds in water over night. Make a paste of the seeds using water. Apply the paste directly on your scalp and give it a rest for 20 minutes. Wash your hair thoroughly with water.

b. Fenugreek Oil and Yogurt:

Ingredients:

4-5 tablespoon Fenugreek Oil

3 tablespoon Yogurt

Process:

Mix fenugreek oil and yogurt and beat them well to make a paste. Apply the paste on your scalp and massage until it is absorbed well. Wash your hair with mild shampoo after wards.

c. Hot Oil Massage

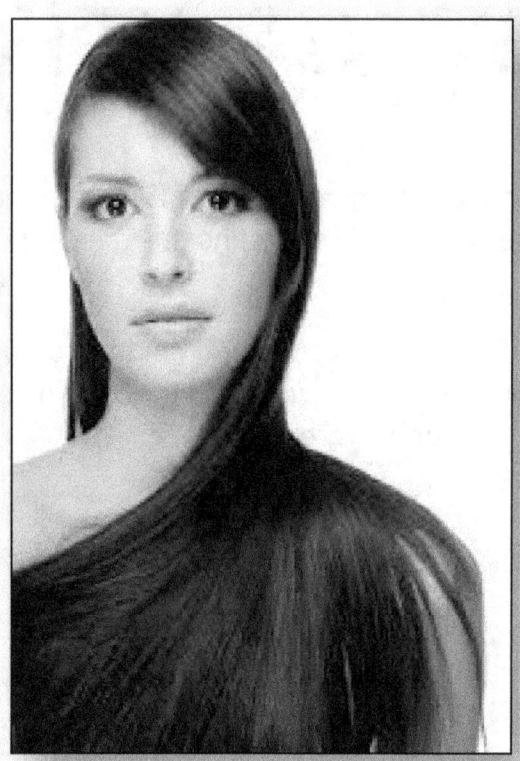

Heat the fenugreek oil. Make sure it is war enough for your scalp to tolerate it. It shouldn't be too warm that it burns your scalp and destroys the layer. Massage your scalp with lukewarm fenugreek oil before going to bed. Wash off your head next morning with a mild shampoo.

d. Fenugreek Leaves and Apple Cider

Ingredients:

1 cup Fenugreek leaves

1 Tablespoon of Apple Cider Vinegar

Water to form a paste

Process:

Wash fenugreek leaves thoroughly with water. Now blend fenugreek leaves apple cider and water together to form a paste with normal consistency. Apply the paste on your scalp one hour before shower. Wash your hair with a mild shampoo. You can apply this remedy 2- times a week for long and string hair.

Potato Juice for Hair Growth

You might not be aware of the wonders of Potato. Not only is this vegetable a part of our daily meal. It can also be used to strengthen your hair. This is not very old remedy. Not many people are familiar with it. Potato has natural starch in it. It helps in making the roots of your hair strong.

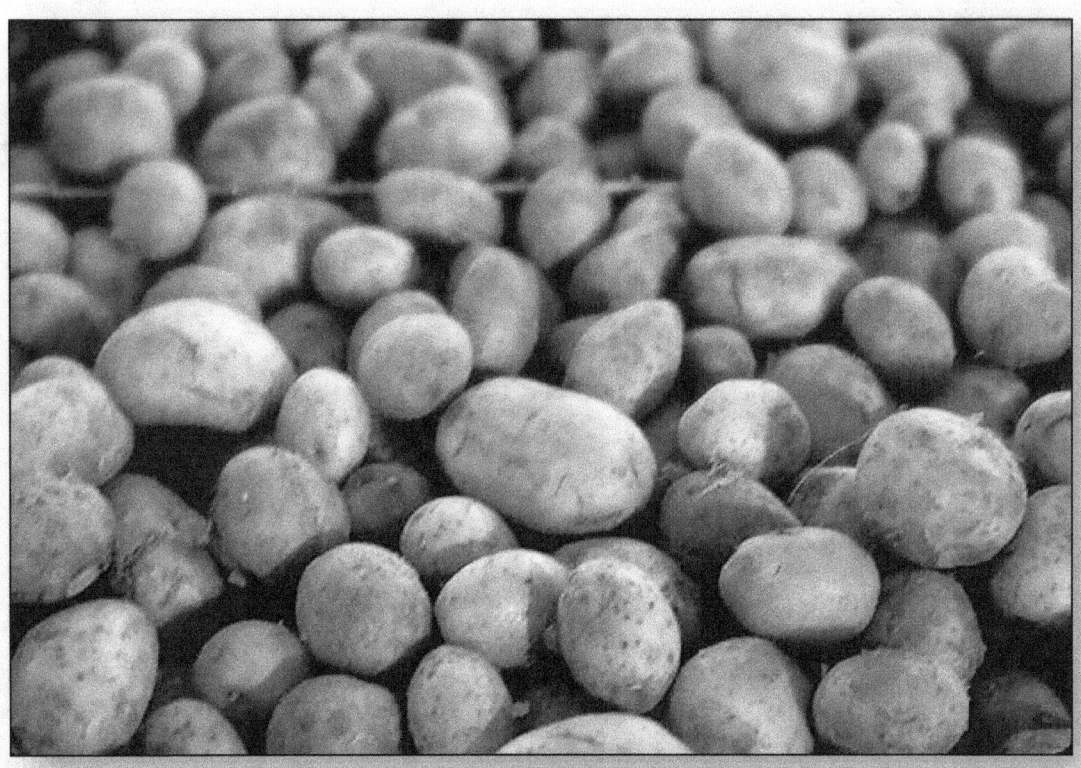

How to Make Potato Juice

Chop Potatoes into small cubes and blend them into water. The potatoes if blend rightly will start to look like a puree. It will be too thick, add a little water in it and blend well. Put it aside for 20 minutes. Strain the puree and separate water from the remnants of potato. Now you have the juice of potato, ready to be used.

Remedies

a. *Potato Juice for Hair*

Ingredients:

½ glass potato juice

Process:

Apply potato juice in your like a tonic and massage well. Repeat the process until all of the potato juice has been used. Absorb the juice in your scalp by massaging your hair constantly. Wash your hair with lukewarm water and if the need be then wash your hair with shampoo.

b. *Potato Juice, Honey and Egg Mask for Hair*

Ingredients:

½ glass Potato Juice

2 tablespoon of Honey

1Egg Yolk

Process:

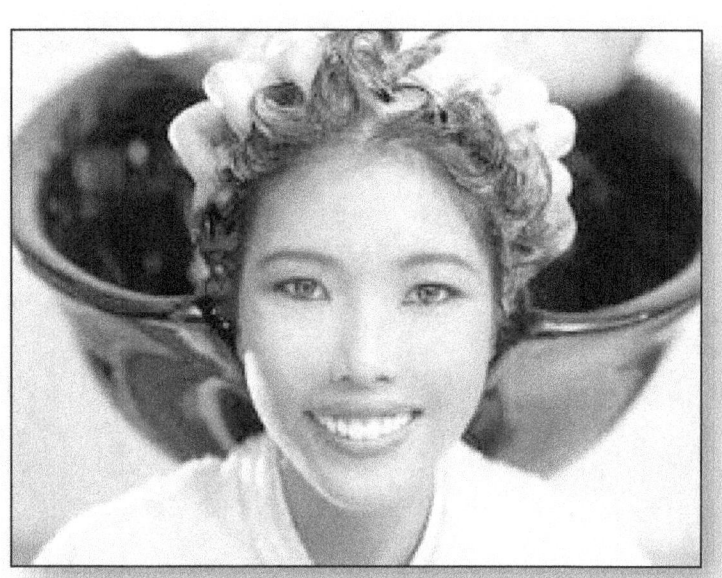

Mix well all the ingredients in a clean bowl and form a uniform consistency solution. Apply all the mixture on your head like a shampoo and massage well. Give it a rest for

20 minutes and then wash your hair thoroughly. Use a good fruit shampoo to wash your hair and get rid of the smell after wards.

Potato juice will help in strengthening your hair where as honey and egg yolk provides the nourishment that hair requires for growth. Egg yolk is also very effective to prevent hair loss.

Henna Powder for Shiny Hair

Henna is one great herb that has been a part of hair conditioning and coloring from as long one can remember. Henna can be used an excellent hair dye. The peculiar smell and the long lasting effect henna has on hair and its health naturally without any chemical is what makes it personal favorite of men and women alike.

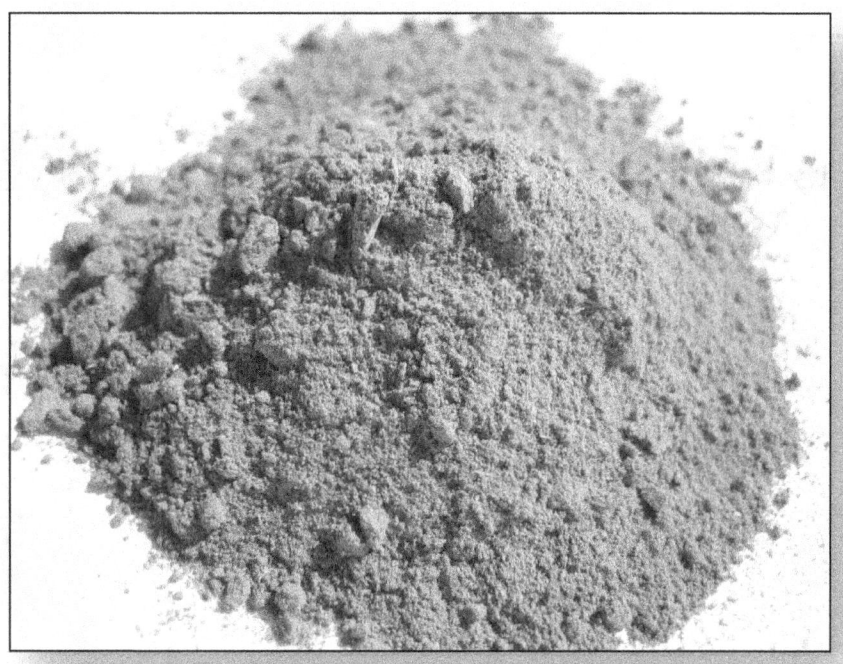

The hair dyes and conditioners available in the market use harsh chemicals and products that damage the keratin layer of your hair and causes pre mature graying of hair. However that is not the case with Henna. Henna act as a great hair dye, the color stays longer than the chemical hair dyes and it also strengthen and conditions your hair giving them natural gloss and shine that no other hair color can.

Remedies:

a. Henna and Honey

Ingredients:

2 Tablespoon of Henna Powder

2 Tablespoon of Honey

Water (To make a paste)

Process:

Mix well all the ingredients and make a thick paste. If you don't want to color hair then apply the mixture immediately. Allow the mixture to dry; it will take approximately 1-2 hours. You can wear a plastic cap around your head to prevent the mixture from dripping and creating a mess.

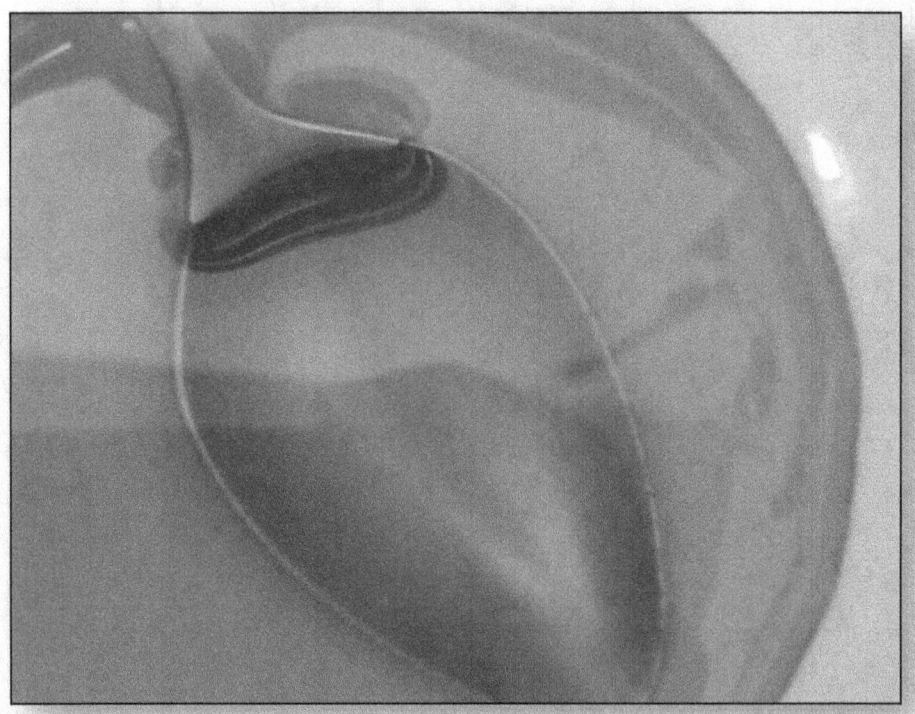

Wash your head under the running water. Thoroughly rinse your hair and get the dried henna mixture out of your head. Henna combined with honey makes your hair soft and shiny. But if you feel your hair is a bit dry then you can apply conditioner after washing your hair.

b. Henna, Tea and Coffee for Conditioning and Coloring

Ingredients:

4 tablespoon of Henna

¼ cup of Tablespoon of strong tea essence.

2-3 tablespoon of coffee essence

2 Tablespoon of Honey as moisturizer

Process:

Mix all the ingredients and form a thick paste. Keep aside the mixture. Henna powder takes time to release its color. By making a paste with tea and coffee essence, it allows Henna to result dark brown color.

Apply the mixture in your hair using a brush. Always wear gloves to prevent nails and hands from getting stained. Leave the mixture in your hair for one or two hours then wash your hair thoroughly under a running tap water. Apply any conditioner after washing your hair if your feel they are a bit dry.

c. Henna and Orange Juice

Ingredients:

3-4 tablespoon of Henna Powder

¼ cup of orange juice

Water

Process:

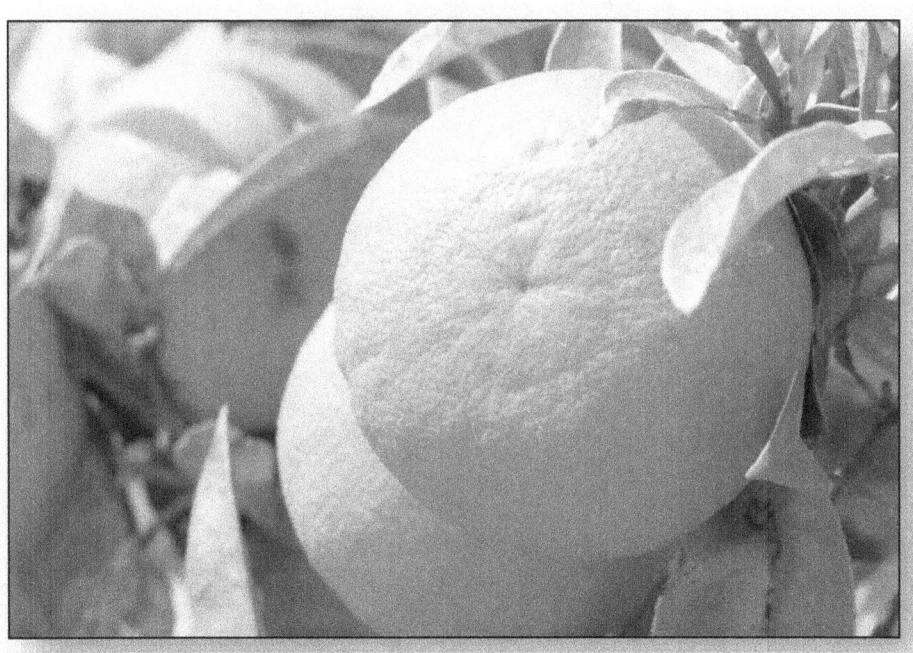

Make a paste of all the ingredients and keep the mixture aside for henna to release its color. If you don't want to color your hair and are only using Henna for strengthening and growing your hair. Then apply the mixture immediately.

Allow the mixture to dry. Then wash your hair thoroughly under running tap water. Henna will strengthen your hair for better growth where as citrus and vitamin C in the orange juice will provide nourishment.

   d. Henna, Shikakai and Gooseberry powder

Ingredients:

2-3 tablespoon of Henna Powder

2-3 Tablespoon of dried Shikakai and Gooseberry Powder

2 Tablespoon of Honey

Water

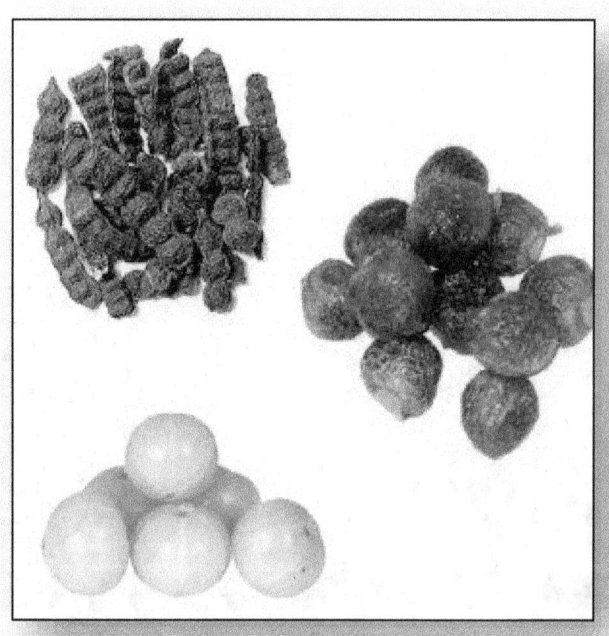

Process:

Mix all the ingredients and form a thick paste. Keep aside the mixture for a couple of hours for henna to release the color if you want to color your hair. Apply the mixture in your hair and wash thoroughly after 1-2 hours.

Henna will give your hair natural gloss and shine, whereas Shikakai and gooseberry powder will strengthen your hair and will make your hair stronger. These ingredients are also very effective when it comes to hair growth.

Aloe Vera for Longer and Stronger Hair

Hair loss is the problem that every second man on this planet is facing for one reason or another. Looking beautiful and charming is wish of every one out their but the emerging problem of excessive hair loss is keeping us from it.

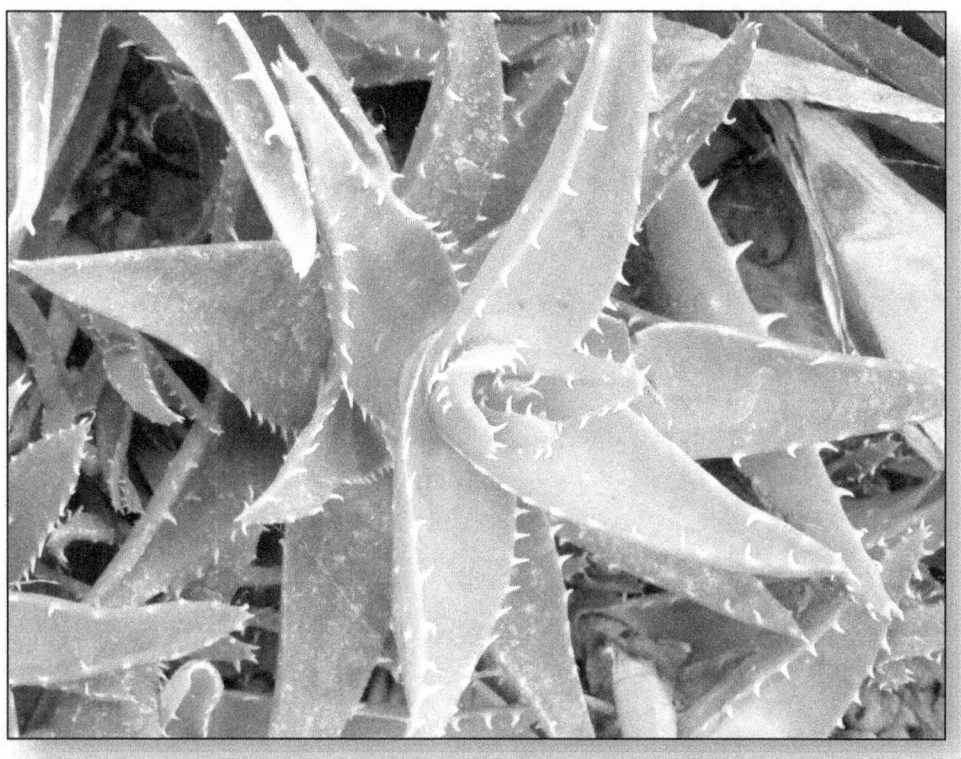

Wouldn't you wish that there was a miracle to cure this issue? Well congratulations, thanks to natural remedies, preventing and curing hair loss is possible. You need to keep in mind few ingredients that nourish hair from roots to tips. One of those ingredients is Aloe Vera.

Aloe Vera has the properties that strengthen your hair and helps in hair growth. Following are a couple of tips for you to keep in mind that involves use of Aloe Vera:

Remedies:

a. Aloe Vera Gel For Hair Growth and Strength:

Ingredients:

3-4 Tablespoon of Aloe Vera Gel

Process:

Cut the Aloe Vera leaves into halves and scoop out the gel from the leaves. Scoop out at least 2-3 tablespoon of Aloe gel. Mix some water in the gel, mash it with help of a fork and then apply the gel on your scalp with help of fingertips. Wash your hair after 30-40 minutes with any mild shampoo.

Repeat the process 2-3 days a week for a month and then do it at least once a week. You will see visible results and reduced hair fall in a month.

b. Hibiscus Flower Powder and Aloe Gel for Hair Loss

Ingredients:

2-3 tablespoon of Dry Hibiscus Flower Powder

2-3 tablespoon of Aloe Gel

Water to form a paste

Process:

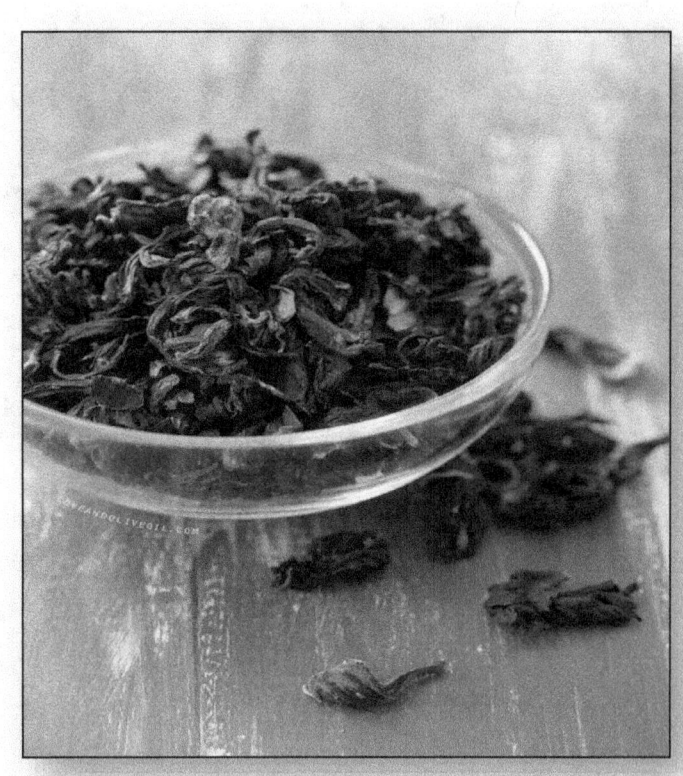

Mix all the ingredients in a clean bowl and form a paste. Mash the Aloe gel with help of a form. Apply the mixture on your scalp and massage thoroughly. Wash your hair after 30-40 minutes with water.

Repeat the process daily for one week. After that you can continue choose to apply it 2-3 times a week. Ale Vera gel will help in hair growth and strength where as Hibiscus flower powder will help in restoring the natural shine of your hair.

   c. Lemon Juice and Aloe Gel for Oily Hair

Ingredients:

2-3 tablespoon of Aloe Vera Gel

2 tablespoon of Lemon Juice

Process:

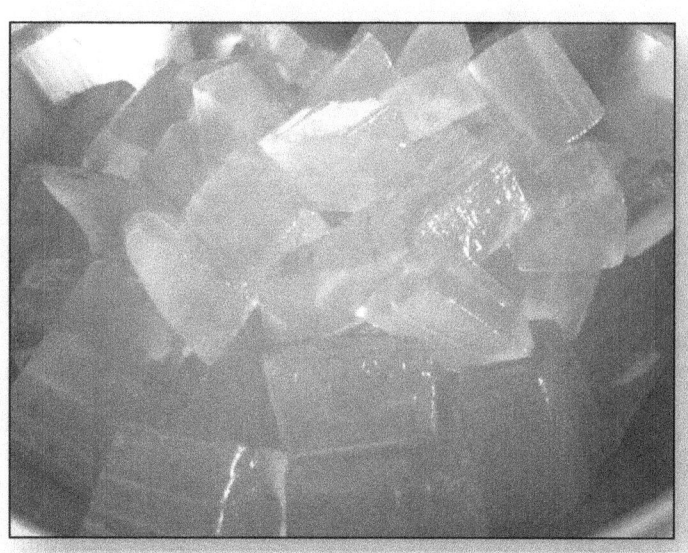

Apply the mixture directly on your scalp and massage your scalp thoroughly. Wash your hair thoroughly with water. Lemon will eliminate the excess oil from your hair and give them natural shine and glow, whereas Aloe Vera will strengthen your hair from roots to tip.

Orange Juice to Get Rid Of the Dandruff and Itchy Scalp

Orange is high in vitamin C and citrus. These two elements are extremely essential when it come s to hair growth. Orange juice not only helps in hair growth but its acerbic properties helps in the removal of excess oil and grease from your hair.

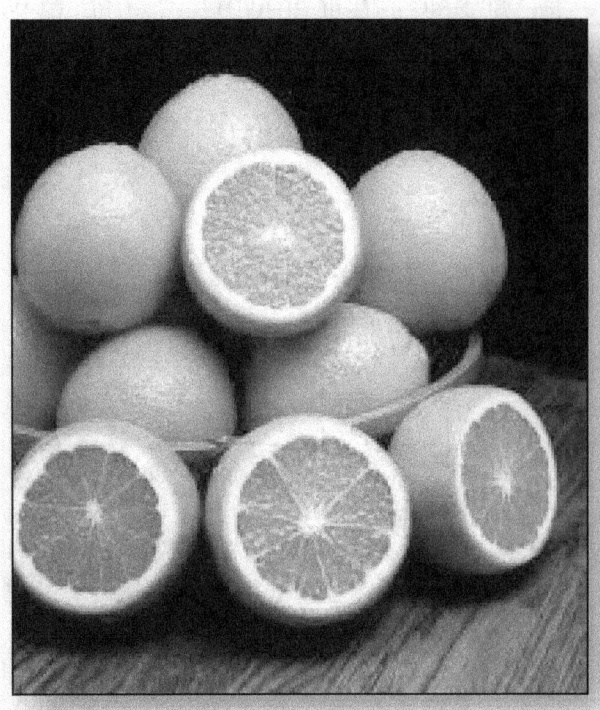

Remedies:

a. Apple and Orange Juice Tonic for Hair Growth

Ingredients:

¼ cup of Orange Juice

¼ cup of Apple juice

½ tablespoon of Apple Cider Vinegar

Process:

Add all the ingredients in a spray bottle and shake well. Spray the mixture on your roots. Then massage your scalp thoroughly. Allow the mixture to settle in the roots. Wash your hair after 30-40 minutes with plain water.

Orange juice and apple will provide the nourishment to your hair as well as strengthen them. Apple Cider vinegar will remove the access oil from your scalp and will give your hair natural shine and gloss.

b. Orange Peel Paste for Hair Growth

Ingredients:

1 Orange Peel

Rose Water to make a paste

Process:

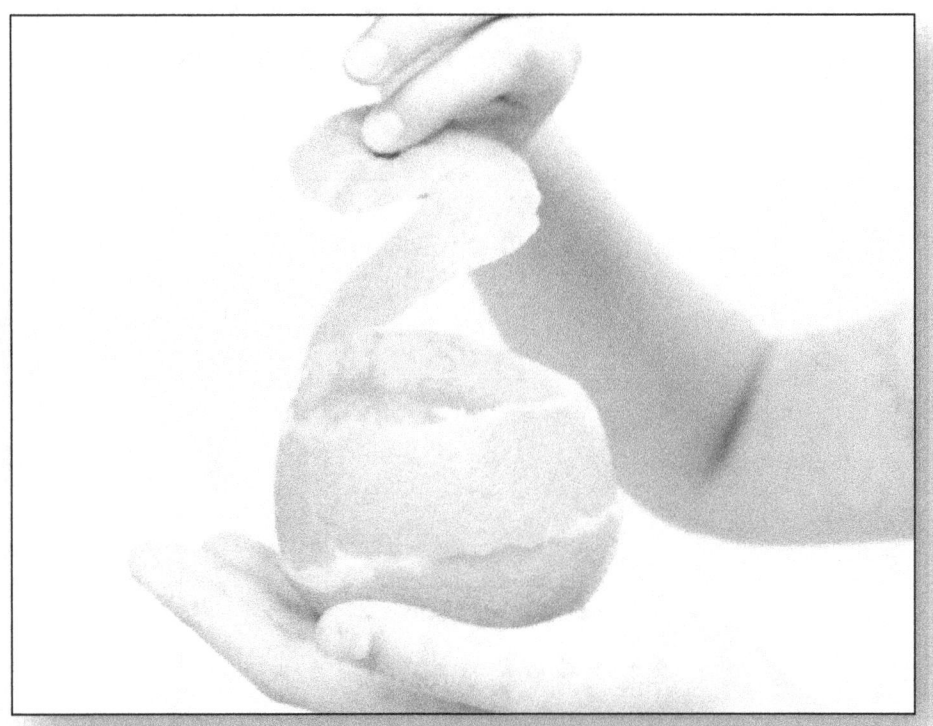

Soak Orange peel in rose water for one hour then mash the peel with help of a fork. Mash it well to turn it into a paste. Add more rose water if needed. Apply the mixture directly to your scalp with help of fingers. Massage your scalp for 5 minutes then allow the mixture to dry. Wash your hair after 30-40 minutes. Comb your hair upside down under running water tap water to get the particles of orange peel completely out of your hair.

Natural Home Remedies for Flawless Skin

You may be a fan of chemical and cosmetics to cure every problem of your skin but did you know these chemical and cosmetics have reactions which can lead to other skin problems like dryness, lack of shine and glow on face. It is, therefore, advised that you opt for natural remedies for your skin. They don't really have side effects, until or unless you are allergic to one or another ingredients being used.

There are several ingredients that are present in your kitchen and you had no idea that they can be used to effectively bring back the glow and shine on your face. Try these simple, easy and natural remedies for natural, flawless and glowing skin.

Baking Soda to Get Rid of the Blemish Scars

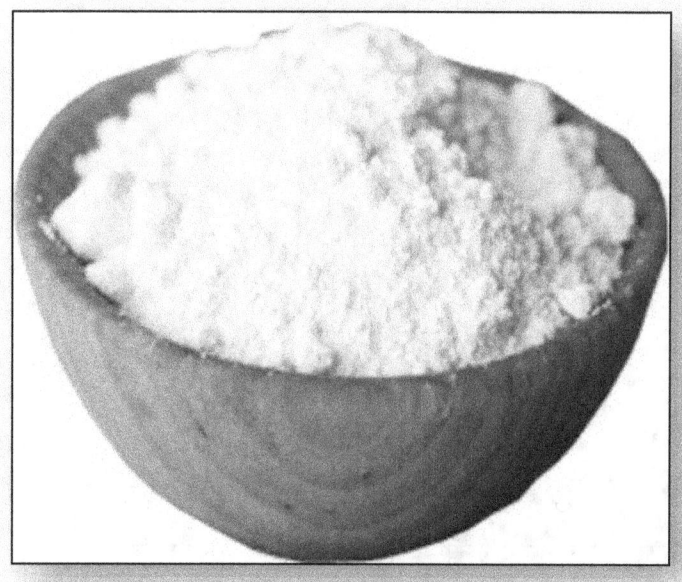

Baking soda has many uses. You might be a fan of the ingredient due to its results in baking but you will be amazed to know what wonders this ingredients can do to your Skin. Baking soda can be extremely effective when it comes to removing scars of the blemishes and pimples.

Take one teaspoon of baking soda add few drops of water and mix it with a finger rub the paste on the scars and the pimples gently. And allow the mixture to dry. Wash off your face with plain water. Repeat the process daily for best result. And don't forget natural remedies takes time to show result.

Neem Tree Leaves To Reduce Acne and Blemishes

Neem tree leaves are known for their antiseptic and healing powers. They are being used as an effective remedies for several skin issues from as long as one can remember.

Neem leaves can be used in number of ways to cure pimples and blemishes, especially in your early teens, some kids face severe acne problems due to hormonal imbalance or due to lack of hygiene and care for skin.

Remedies:

Neem Tree Leaves Paste and Oil as a Cure for Blemishes

Neem Oil:

One of the most easiest and effective way to cure blemishes by neem tree is by applying neem oil directly on the pimples and blemishes. It dries out the pimples and gets rid of the painful blemishes in a matter of days.

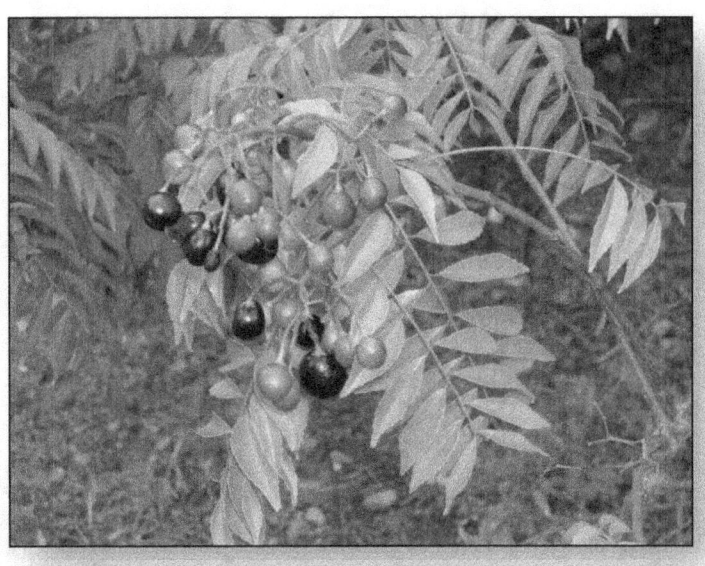

Neem Leaves' Paste:

Make a paste of neem leaves by crushing them in pastel and mortar; add a little water to make a paste. Apply the paste directly on the blemishes, pimples or scars and allow it to dry. It will dry out the pimples and prevent them from leaving marks.

You can apply this remedy daily for best results. Make sure you wash the neem leaves thoroughly before making a paste.

Milk and Cucumber Mask to Get Rid of the Oily Skin and Blemishes

Milk and cucumber are two ingredients that are present in our fridge all the time and are easily available at the nearest grocery store without any hassle. To the surprise of many these two ingredients can be of great use if you want to cure your oily skin and blemishes that result due to the excessive oil on your skin.

Here is how you can use these simple ingredients to cure the problem you have been long trying to get rid of.

Remedy:

a. Milk and Cucumber Mask For Blemishes and Oil Control:

Take one cucumber and cut it into pieces. Blend the cucumber with just enough amount of milk to make a paste. When the mixture is of uniform consistency pour it out into a clean bowl. Apply the paste all over your face and give it a rest for 30 minutes and then wash your face thoroughly with water.

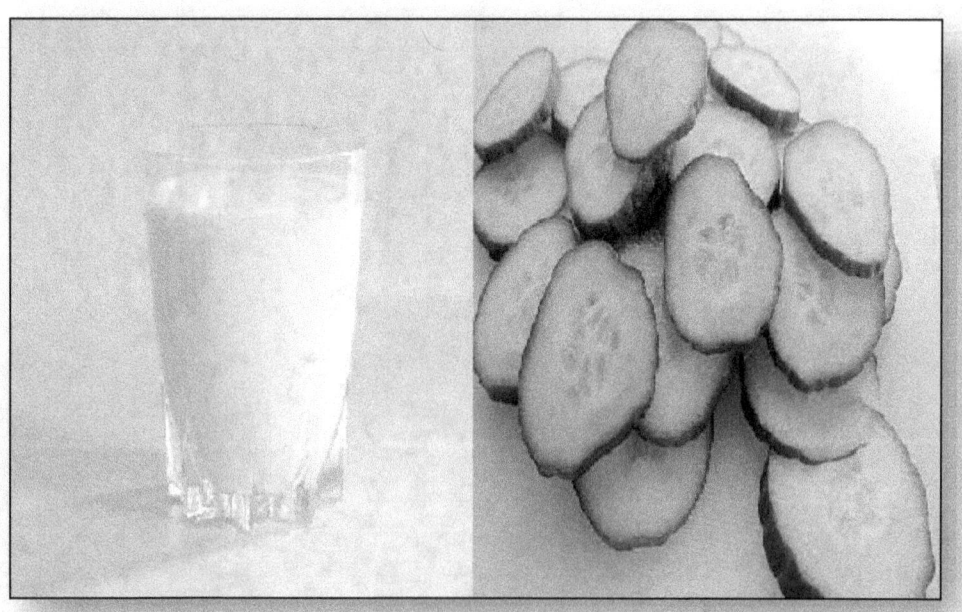

b. Cucumber Toner for Oil Control:

Blend one cumber with half cup of water. Filter water from the cumber by using linen cloth. Fill the water in a spray bottle and apply it on your face multiple times a day. Don't wipe the tonic. One cucumber is enough to make a tonic enough for use of a day. Make sure you make fresh tonic every day.

Honey Treatment to Get Rid of the Dark Spots and Blemishes:

Honey is being used in several beauty products from ancient times. Women and men have been a fan of the miracles honey has to offer. From having antiseptic properties to weight reduction capabilities honey has it all. You can even use honey to reduce dark spots from your skin and it also helps in preventing the blemishes by exfoliating your skin from the pores.

Remedies:

Honey and Lemon to Cure Dark Spot and Prevent Blemishes:

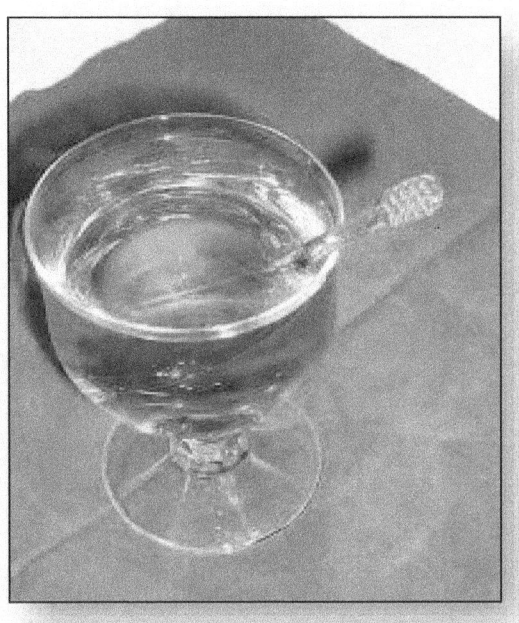

Take 1 table spoon of Honey and add one tablespoon of lemon juice to it. Mix well and add rose water if you think the mixture is a bit thick. Apply the mixture on the blemishes and allow it to dry. It will dry out the blemish and prevent from leaving marks.

You can also apply this mixture on your nose and cheek. Allow it dry and then clean your face by washing it with plain water. Honey will remove the dead cell from your skin and prevent the blemishes from growing.

Apply the mixture on the areas with dark spots and patches. Honey will reduce the patches on your skin.

Turmeric Powder and Milk Cream to Lighten Your Skin Tone

Several cosmetic products and creams have been advertising about turmeric and milk cream as the ingredient of their whitening and skin lightening creams but we all know natural ingredients applied directly without any chemical intervention, works best.

Remedies:

Turmeric, Saffron and Milk Cream

Ingredients:

Pinch of Turmeric Powder

Pinch of Saffron

2Tablespoon of Milk Cream

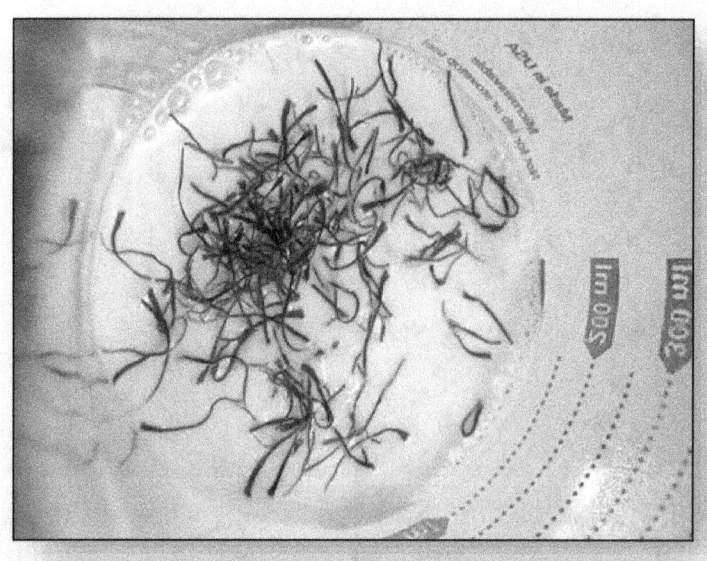

Process:

Add all the ingredients in a clean bowl and mix well until the milk cream slightly changes the color. Apply this mixture all over your face and massage gently for five minutes. Allow the mask/paste to then dry on your face. Wipe of the remnants with help of the cotton balls. Wash your face thoroughly with water or any mild face wash.

Mud Mask to reduce Oil from Face

If you are not allergic to natural products like Fuller's Earth and other mud then you will be extremely delighted to know that mud masks are highly effective in unclogging your pores, reducing oil from your skin a s a result and also have numerous other benefits including skin tightening and reducing aging signs.

Remedies:

Fuller's Earth Mask

Ingredients:

2 Tablespoon of Fuller's Earth

Rose Water to make a paste

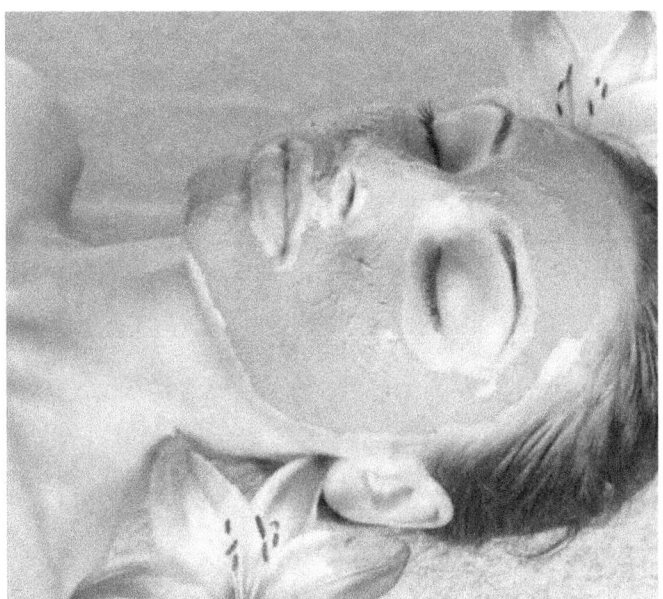

Process:

Usually Fuller's earth is in the form of blocks you can even soak the blocks over night and then use it the next day. Make a paste of Fuller's earth in rose water and apply it on your face. Apply upward stroke. Allow the mask to dry on your face. When it is completely dry and scaly, wash your face with water massage thoroughly.

Cabbage Toner and Green Tea to Reduce Oil on Skin

You cannot deny the part that a good toner plays in oil controlling and making your face look fresh. You can prepare your own toner at home with all natural ingredients. One of the main benefits of the natural ingredients is that you know there aren't any chemical ingredients that will harm your skin.

Remedies:

Cabbage Toner

Ingredients:

1 Cup Cabbage

2 cup water

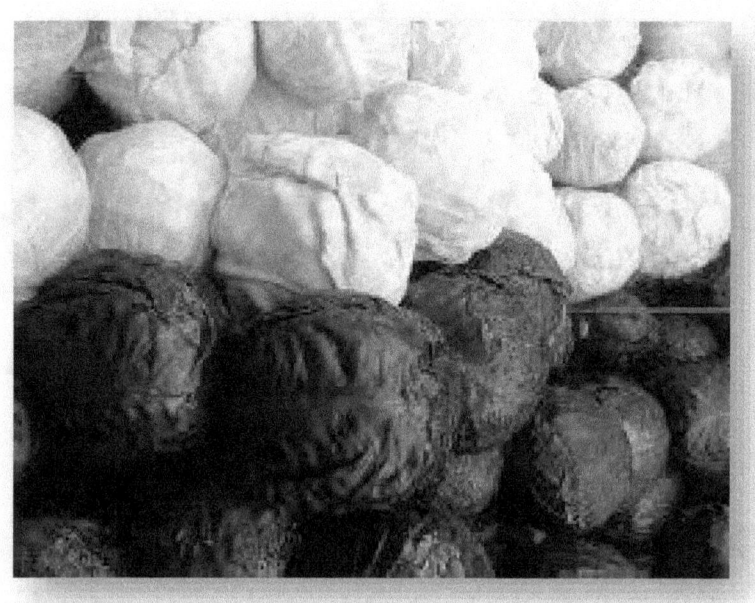

Process:

Boil cabbage in water. When the water changes its color to yellowish-green and cabbage becomes soft. Turn off the stove. Extract the cabbage and put the water aside. Allow it to cool and then fill the water in a spray bottle.

After washing your face, apply this toner and allow it dry. Don't wipe off your face afterwards. This will close your pores and prevent excess oiling of your skin.

Green Tea Toner

Ingredients:

1 tablespoon of Green Tea

1½ cup of water

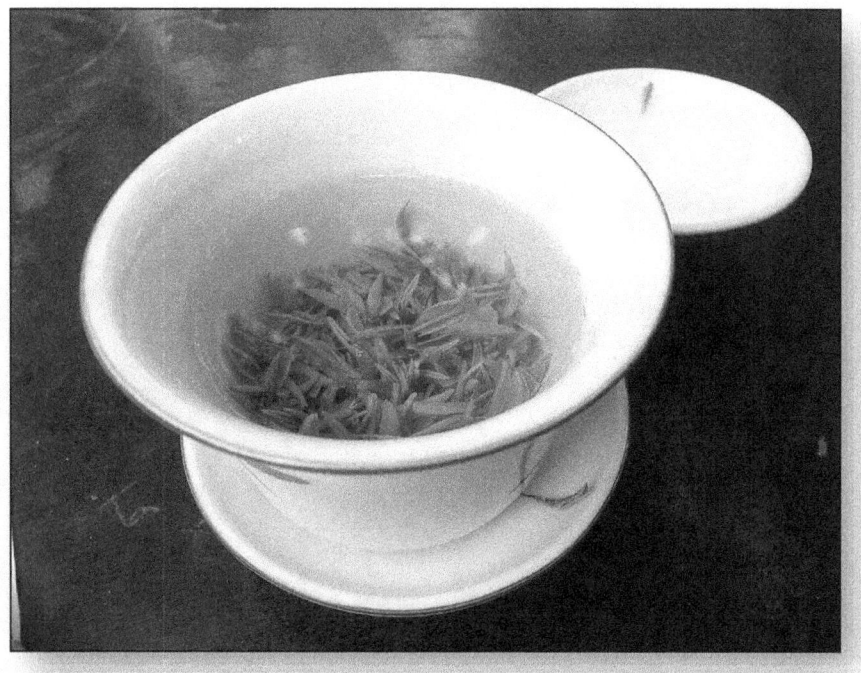

Process:

Boil one and a half cup of water and add green tea to it. Extract the green tea in a bowl and allow it to cool. Pour it in an ice cube tray and freeze it. Use one cube at a time to massage your face after long sun exposure or apply it after washing your face. This will close your pore and prevent excess oil to appear on your face.

Egg White Mask to Reduce Wrinkles

After 25 years of age men and women starts to show signs of aging. The skin starts to lose its elasticity and becomes lose, resulting wrinkles. However you do not have to worry about starting to look old. You can make a natural egg mask that will help you in fighting wrinkles and other signs of aging. The result of this mask lasts longer than the cosmetic masks available in the market.

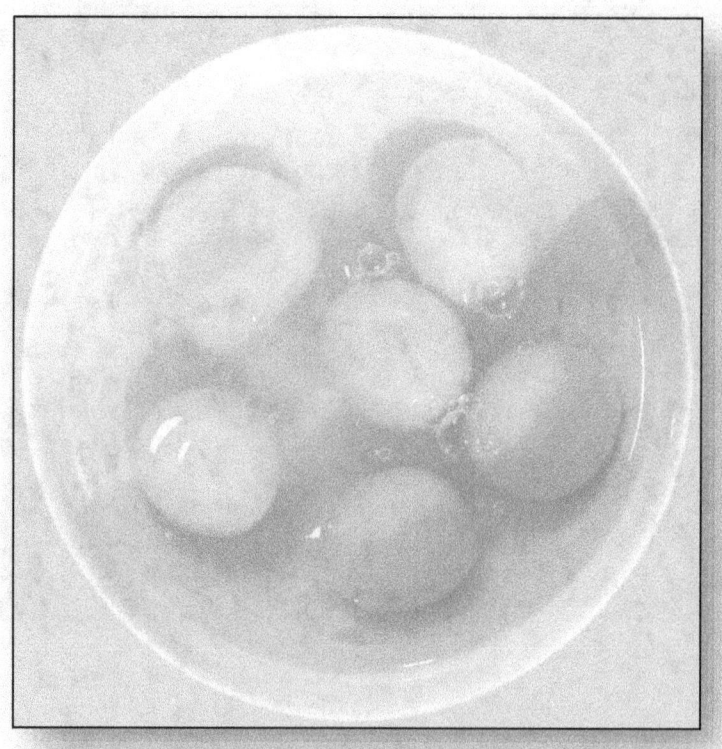

Remedies:

How to Prepare Egg Mask:

Ingredients:

1 Egg

Process:

Beat the egg yolk and white until they are of uniform consistency. Apply the mixture as a mask on your face with help of a brush or fingers. Make sure you apply upward strokes. Allow the mask to dry. Wash your face thoroughly with water afterwards. Spray rose water on your face to get rid of the smell of egg.

Remove Black and Whiteheads with Nutmeg

When it comes to removing blackheads, scrubs with rough particles helps in unclogging pores and removing blackheads. It is advised to scrub your face 2-3 times a week. But the amount of chemical products they use in the scrubs available in the market, it is not likely to use scrub 2-3 times a week.

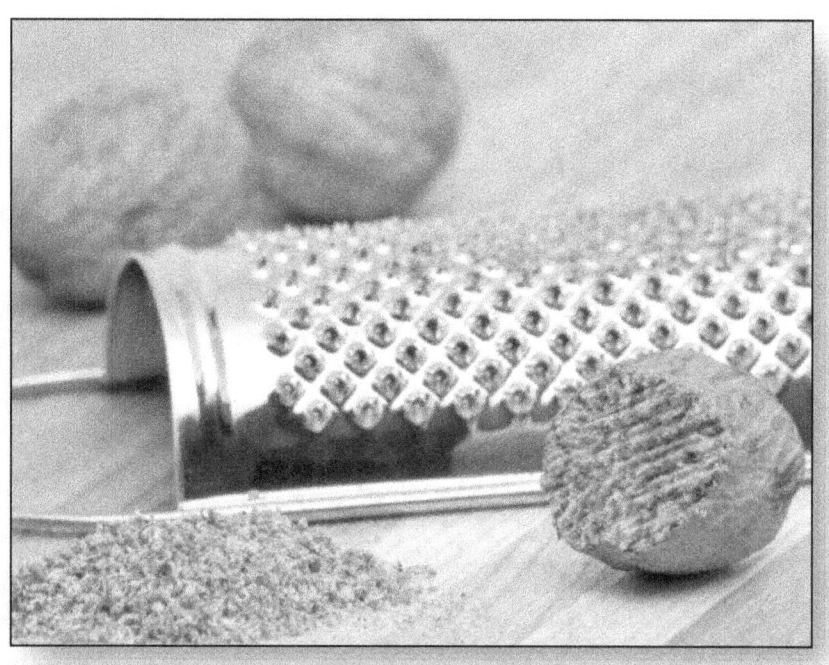

Remedies

Nutmeg Paste

Ingredients:

2 tablespoon of Nutmeg

Rose water to make a paste

Process:

Take nutmeg powder in a bowl and add enough rosewater to make a thick paste. Apply it on your nose, cheeks and chin. Scrub gently for 3-4 minutes. Apply the rest of the paste on your face and allow it to dry. Wash your face thoroughly with water afterwards.

Tomato Pulp to Remove Whiteheads

Like blackheads, whiteheads are equal trouble makers. White heads are composed of the similar content but they are not oxidized hence white. Removing whiteheads can be very troubling but with help of this one ingredient in your kitchen you will be able to get rid of them naturally, without using any chemical products.

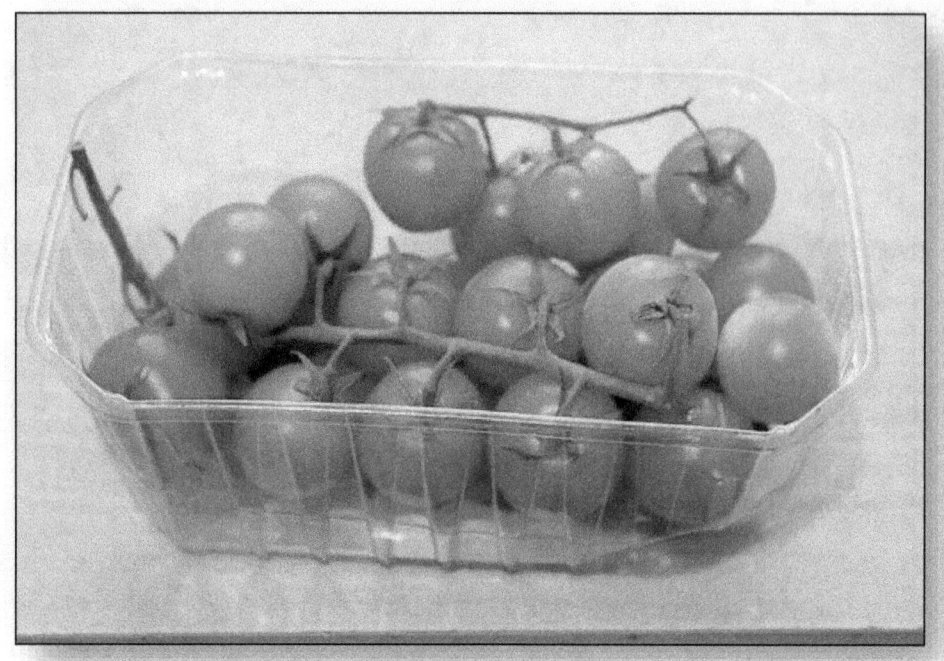

Remedies:

Tomato Paste and Tonic to Cure Whiteheads

Ingredients:

1 tomato

2 tablespoon of witch hazel

Water to make a paste

Process:

Blend all the ingredients and make a puree. Apply just enough puree to massage your face with it. Massage your face for 2-3 minutes. Apply rest of the mixture on your face and leave it for 1015 minutes, depending upon the time you have. Wash your face thoroughly with water.

Banana Mask to Deal with Dry and Patchy Skin

In winters and even usually, most of the people complain about dry patches on skin. These dry patches often cause discoloration of skin. It is best if you treat them on time. Natural remedies with easily available ingredients can help you with this problem.

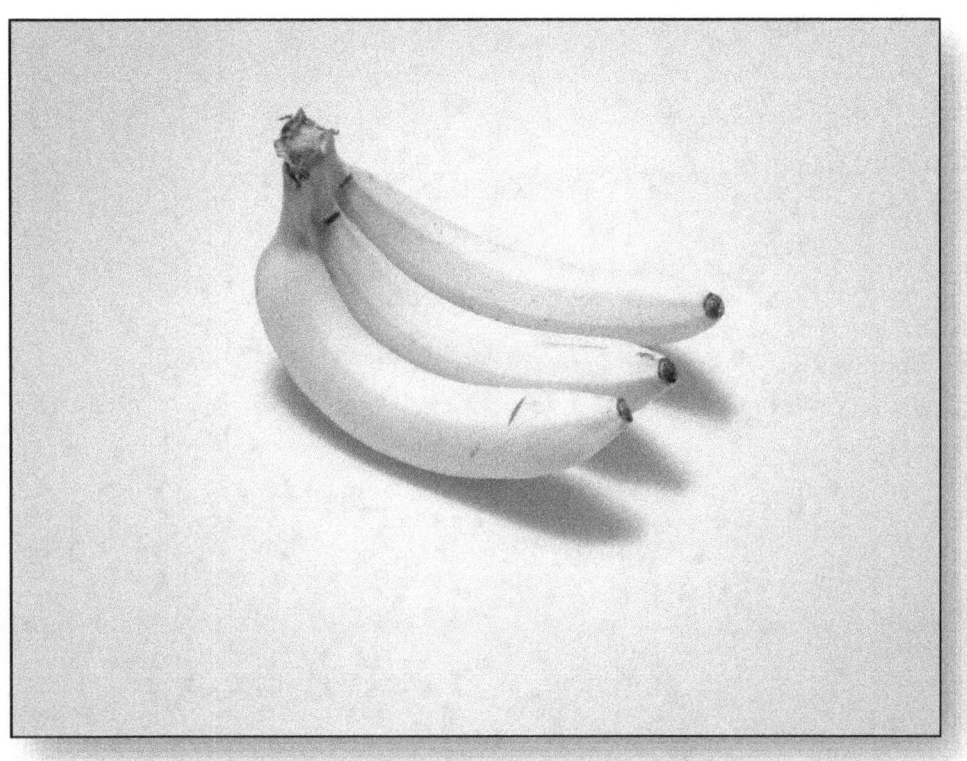

Remedy:

Banana Mask

Ingredients:

1 Banana

2-4 tablespoon of milk

1tablespoon of Honey

Process:

Peel a banana and mash it to pulp with help of a fork. Add honey and milk to it and mash once again to make a paste. Apply the paste on the dry patches on your skin and massage gently. Leave it for 10-20 minutes and then wash the area with water. Apply rose water afterwards.

Use of Shea Butter and Butter Milk to Moisturize Skin

Moisturizing your skin is an essential part of the skin care. It doesn't matter I you have oily or dry skin. Every skin requires moisturizing to look supple, fresh and hydrated. The amount of moisturizing, however, depends upon your skin type. You can prepare your own natural moisturizer at home which will not only moisturize your skin, it has numerous other benefits.

Remedy:

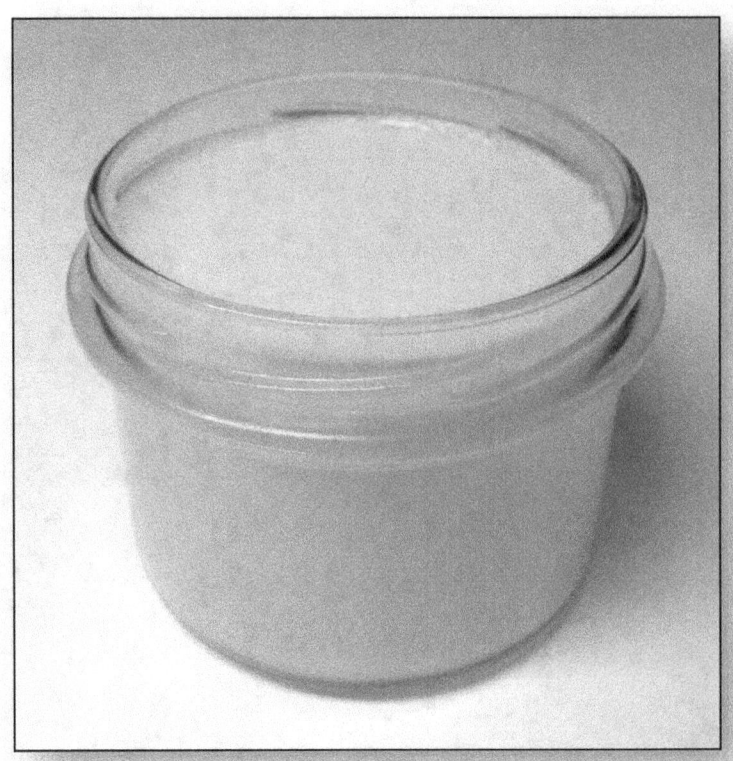

Butter milk and Shea Butter Moisturizer:

Ingredients:

½ cup of Butter Milk

2 tablespoon of Shea Butter

Process:

Take a bowl and add both ingredients in it. Mix well and form a paste. Once the mixture is of uniform consistency, store it in a bottle. Apply the moisturizer on your face, hands and feet with help of a cotton ball, or as the need be. You will see visible results right after the first use.

Natural Home Remedies for Maintaining a Fit and Beautiful Body

Having a good physique and attractive features the need of the time. You don't need to be perfect. All you need to do is make yourself appear presentable, your skin glowing and perfect, and keep your body weight in check.

There are several natural remedies around you, if you add them in your life you can manage to live a healthy life. Here are some remedies given for you to make your body look beautiful and represent you in the way you want it to.

Apricot and Avocado Scrub for Natural Shine on Body

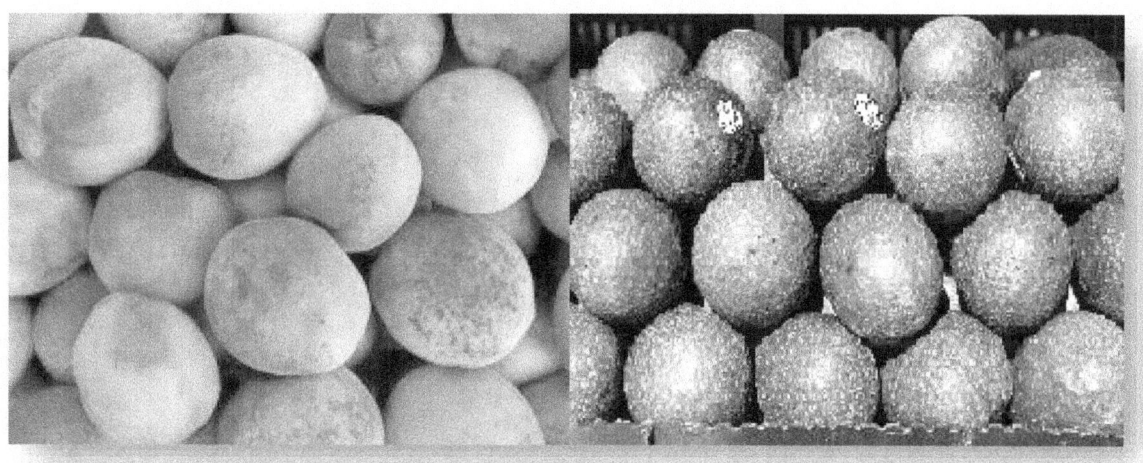

Scrubs helps in removing dead cells and skin from the body and leaves your skin smooth and shiny. Therefore body scrubs and massages are in demand when it comes to body polish and shine. The scrub requirements vary according to skin type however you can use avocado scrub for making your skin smooth and shiny.

Remedies:

Apricot and Avocado Scrub Made at Home:

Ingredients:

1 cup Kernel of Apricot

1 cup Kernel of Avocado

3 tablespoon of Butter milk (If you have dry skin)

1 tablespoon of Shea butter (If you have dry skin)

2 tablespoon of Olive Oil

½ cup fresh Avocado and Apricot paste

Process:

Dry the kernel or seeds of apricot and avocado. When they are completely dried, crush them and make sure you don't leave any sharp corner left. Crush them until they start to look more like a powder. Remove any huge pieces that cannot be further crushed and store the powder in a jar.

For each use take 2 tablespoon of Olive Oil, half cup fresh Avocado and Apricot paste. Add 3 tablespoon of Butter milk and 1 tablespoon of Shea butter if you have dry skin. Make a mixture and apply it on your hands and feet and face if you feel the need of it. Massage well. Leave it on your skin for 10 minutes and then take a bath and wash yourself thoroughly.

Quinoa to Oxidize blood and Reduce Excess Weight

Quinoa is an herb that is used in several Asian foods. However, Quinoa is used all over the world as an ingredient that is known for providing energy, reducing weight and oxidizing blood at the same time. This little wonder has several benefits on our health and body.

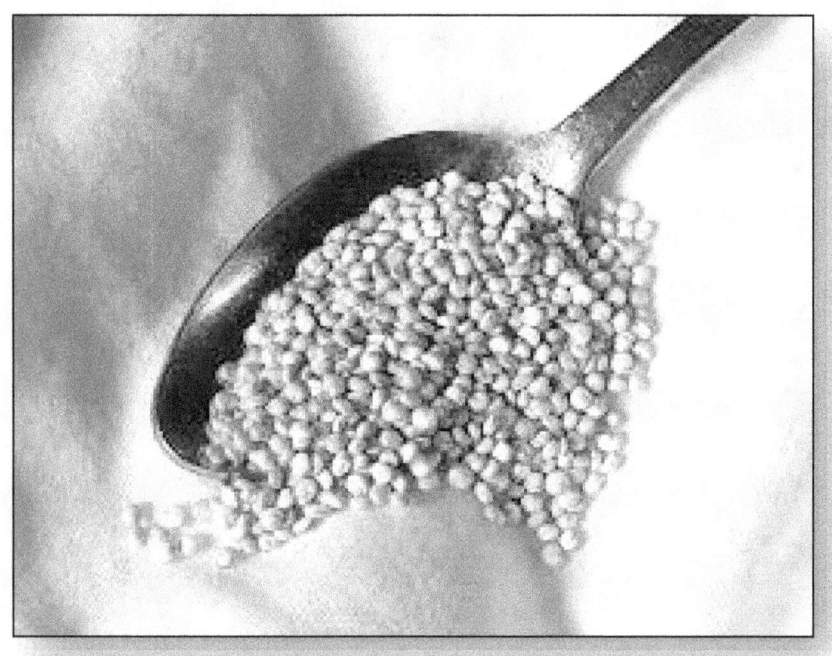

Remedy:

Quinoa Tea

Ingredients:

½ tablespoon of Quinoa

1 ½ cup of water

1 teaspoon of lemon

Process:

Boil water in a saucepan. Add Quinoa to it and then boil one more time. Filter out the quinoa and pour the water in a cup. Add lemon juice to it. You can drink this tea 2 times a day. This will not only oxidize your blood, but will also help you in reducing weight. It provides you enough energy that you get from a full meal.

Use of Honey and Lemon to Keep Your Body Weight in Check

Use of honey and lemon is a part of home based remedies for reducing weight from quite a long time. But little did you know that it has numerous other benefits that make it only fitting to make it a morning ritual to have lemon and honey tea every morning.

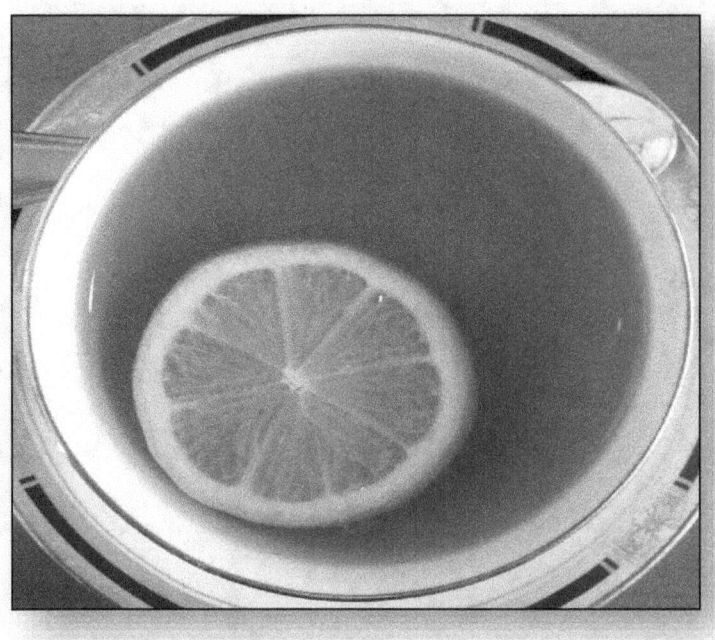

Remedy:

Lemon and Honey Tea

Ingredients:

1 tablespoon of Lemon

1 teaspoon of honey

Process:

Pour boiling hot water in a glass and add 1 tablespoon of lemon and half teaspoon of honey. Dissolve honey in it and wait for the Lemon and Honey tea to get a bit warm. Drink the lukewarm solution, early in the morning before eating anything.

This remedy will cleanse your system, oxidize your blood and will help you in reducing weight. If you have constipation, this remedy is highly effective in that case as well.

Oatmeal to Reduce Cholesterol and Living a Healthy and Fit life

Oatmeal are high in fiber and you must have heard of people who have dramatically reduces weight by oatmeal. Oats absorbs the cholesterol and fats from your body and helps you in reducing weight. They provide you enough energy to carry on your daily routine without any hassle.

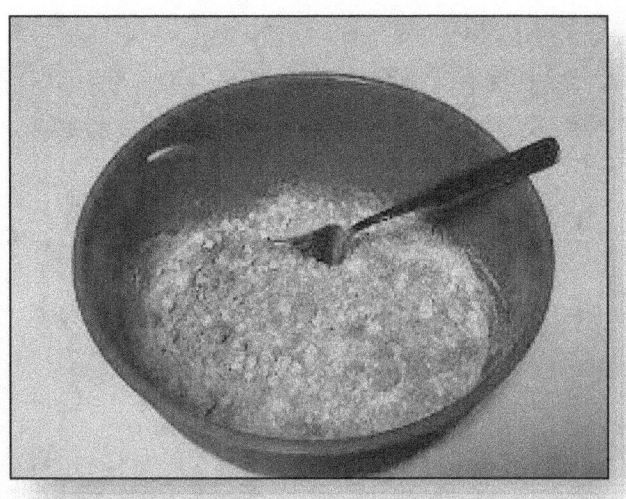

Remedies:

a. Oat Meal, Honey and Pumpkin

Ingredients:

2-3tablespoon full of Oatmeal

1 Cup Water

1 tablespoon of Honey

1cup Pumpkin cut into cubes

Process:

Boil oats in water when they are almost like a porridge, add honey in it. Mix well and take it off of the stove. Add pumpkin cubes in it and coat them well in the porridge. You can eat this cold or hot as per your liking.

b. Oat Meal Yogurt and Raspberries

Ingredients:

2-3 tablespoon of Oatmeal

1cup Water

2tablespoon of Yogurt

1Cup of raspberries

Process:

Boil oats in water when they are almost like porridge add yogurt in it and mix well Add salt and pepper to season and take it off of the stove. Pour the porridge in a bowl and add raspberries on top after it gets cooled down. You can enjoy your meal. Remember it is all about creating your own flavor.

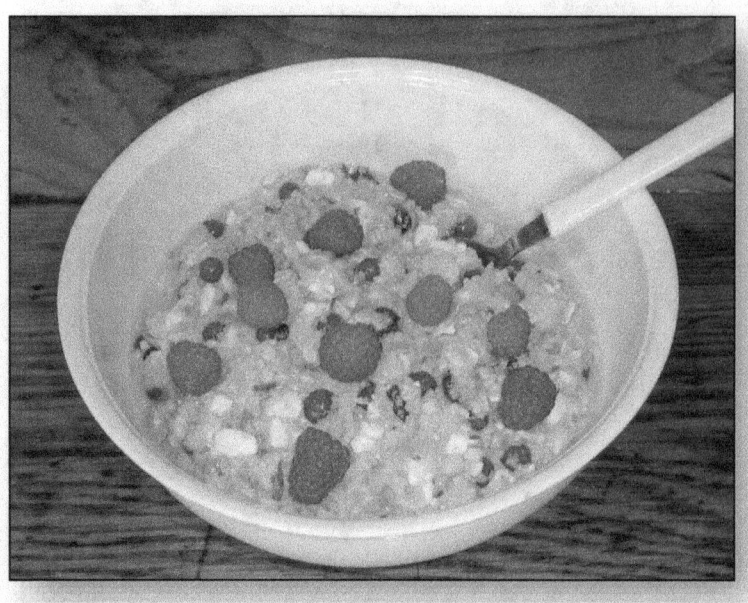

c. Oat Meal, Coconut and Milk

Ingredients:

2-3 tablespoon of Oatmeal

1cup of Skimmed Milk

1 Tablespoon of dried coconut

Process:

Boil oatmeal in milk. Keep stirring until it starts to look like porridge. Add dried coconut to it and your porridge is ready to eat.

Use of Olive Oil to Reduce Weight

Olive oil can help you in curing patchy, dry skin. It can help you in controlling your cholesterol level, reducing weight and what not. Olive oil has numerous advantages. You Will be extremely interested to know that how can you reduce weight by adding this blessing in your life and reduce weight. Olive oil increases your metabolism rate and as a result reduces your weight and control cholesterol.

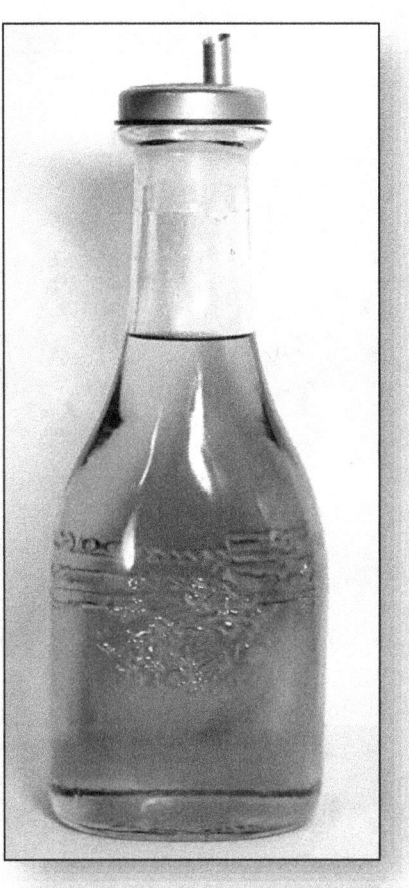

Remedy

Olive Oil an Active Weight Reducing Agent

All you need to do is replace your cooking oil with Olive oil. Olive oil has zero calories and it will increase your metabolism rate and help in digestion. One of the main characteristic features of Olive oil is that it converts the insoluble LDL to HDL which helps in cholesterol and weight reduction. It is not a magic, you will however, have to exercise along with all these tips and remedies to keep yourself in shape.

Adding A Little Cinnamon to Keep the Body in Shape

There are a number of natural ways by which you can reduce weight without any side effects. One of those natural ways is using cinnamon to keep your body in shape. Then if you like the flavor and fragrance of cinnamon, you will enjoy this quick and easy remedy to keep excess weight at bay

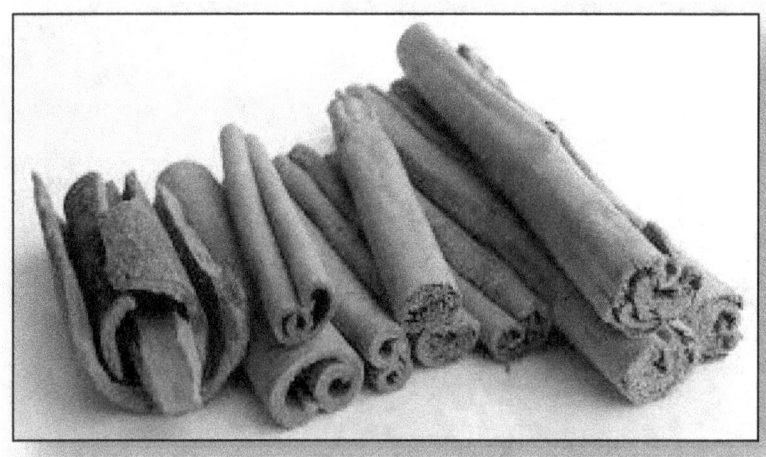

Remedy

Cinnamon Tea:

Ingredients:

1 cinnamon twig

1 cup Water

Process:

Boil a cup of water and add a cinnamon stick to it. Boil until the cinnamon leaves its flavor in the water. You can add more than one cinnamon stick if you like strong flavor. Remove the sticks from water. Add some honey to the Cinnamon tea and enjoy.

You can drink one cup a day. This will not only prevent you from gaining weight but is also very effective for diabetic patients. It controls their blood-sugar level.

Use of Cabbage for Flat Tummy

Cabbage is one natural ingredient that is known for reducing belly fat and making it flat. If you are worried about your pot belly and even after exercise sessions several hours a day you are not able to reduce belly aft than this natural remedy will help you in getting rid of it.

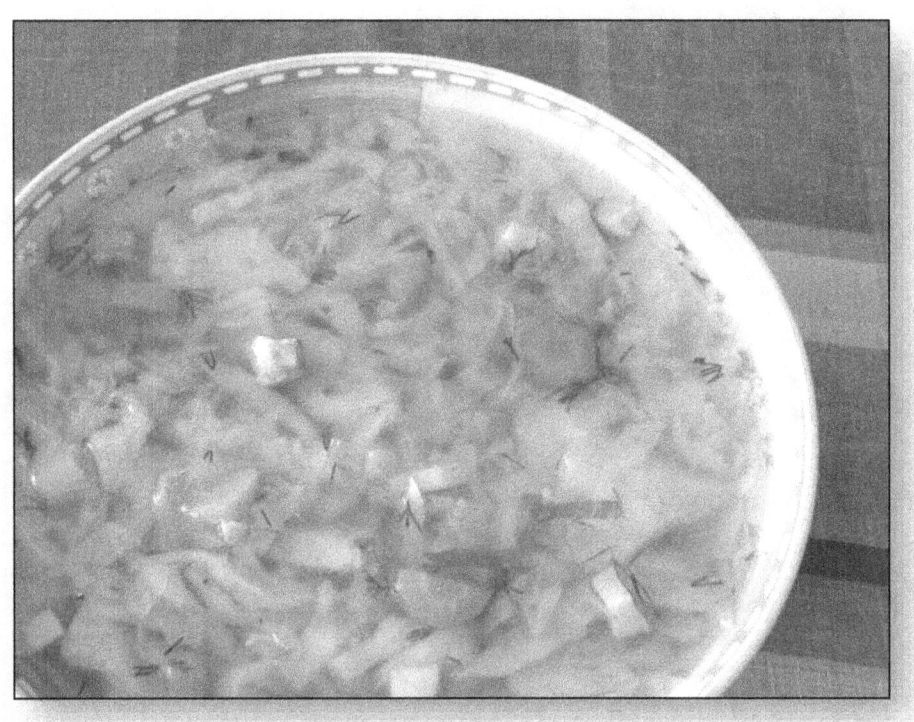

Remedy:

Cabbage Soup to Reduce

Ingredients:

1cup cabbage chopped in square

2 ½ cup of water

Process:

Boil water in sauce pan and add cabbage to it. Boil them for 5-6 minutes. Add salt and pepper to the soup, you can add other spices according to your taste. Drink the soup and you can even eat the cabbage.

Add this soup to your daily diet routine and within one week you will see visible difference in your weight, especially in your belly fat.

Water Melon Diet to Keep Those Extra Pounds Away

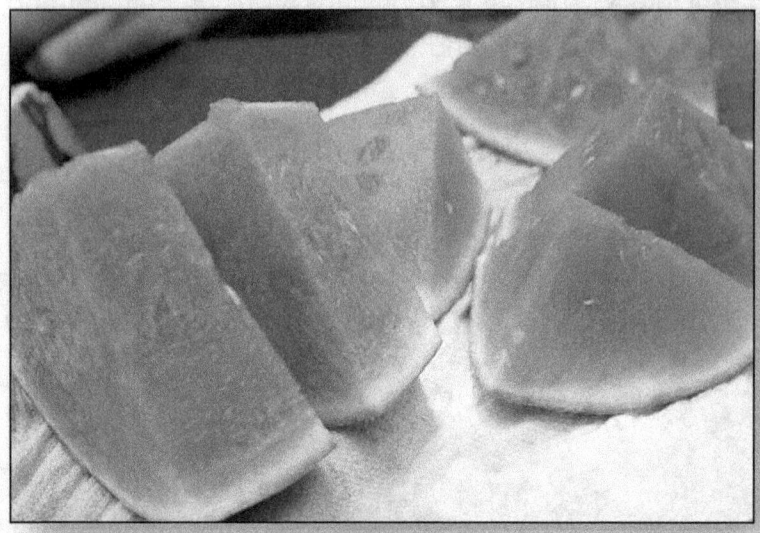

Water Melon is a very tasty fruit. It is so light and refreshing that in summer season you can even replace your lunch or breakfast with watermelon. It refreshes you and is an equivalent of one time meal. But did you know that many people are using this fruit to reduce weight the natural way without any side effects? Now you can do that too. Watermelon is high in glucose and it replaces your meal without making your feel weary.

Remedy:

Watermelon to Effectively Lose Weight

Ingredients:

1 cup water melon (Cut into cubes and seeds removed)

Process:

Eat water melon in breakfast or in brunch. Make sure that you do not eat watermelon after eating anything. It is advised that you consume it empty stomach. After eating watermelon you will not feel the need of eating anything else. It will fulfill your nutritional needs of one time meal and will also help in effectively reducing your weight.

Conclusion:

When it comes to maintaining a good body, skin, hair and over-all health, it is best that you don't rely on chemical based products and opt for natural remedies. These remedies use natural products and derive benefits from them to ensure your problem is solved.

Unlike chemical based beauty and weight reducing products, they don't have adverse effects on our body. While opting for all natural home remedies you need to always keep I n mind that natural remedies takes their time to show result. But in the long run will be extremely beneficial.

Always make sure that you are not allergic to any of the nature; herb, fruit or ingredient. Consult a doctor before following any tip if you are not sure.